Home Care for the Stroke Patient: Living in a Pattern

Margaret Johnstone MCSP

Illustrated by
Estrid Barton

SECOND EDITION

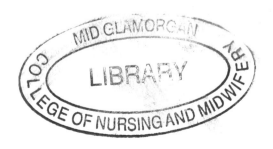

D1514354

CHURCHILL LIVINGSTONE
EDINBURGH LONDON MELBOURNE AND NEW YORK 1987

CHURCHILL LIVINGSTONE
Medical Division of Longman Group UK Limited

Distributed in the United States of America by
Churchill Livingstone Inc., 1560 Broadway, New
York, N.Y. 10036, and by associated companies,
branches and representatives throughout the world.

First edition 1980
Second edition 1987

ISBN 0-443-03399-4

British Library Cataloguing in Publication Data
Johnstone, Margaret
   Home care for the stroke patient: living
   in a pattern. — 2nd ed.
   1. Cerebrovascular disease — Patients —
   Home care
   I. Title   II. Barton, Estrid
   649.8   RC388.5

Library of Congress Cataloging in Publication Data
Johnstone, Margaret.
   Home care for the stroke patient.
   Includes bibliographies and index.
   1. Cerebrovascular disease — Patients — Home care.
   2. Cerebrovascular disease — Patients — Rehabilitation.
   I. Title.   [DNLM: 1. Cerebrovascular Disorders —
   rehabilitation — popular works.   2. Home Nursing.
   WL 355 J73h]
   RC388.5.J617   1986   649.8   86-9553

Produced by Longman Group (FE) Ltd
Printed in Hong Kong

Preface

Home Care for the Stroke Patient: Living in a Pattern has been written as a necessary follow up to my previous books on the care of the stroke patient.

The Stroke Patient: Principles of Rehabilitation was written chiefly for nurses. *Restoration of Motor Function in the Stroke Patient* was written chiefly for physiotherapists.

Home Care for the Stroke Patient: Living in a Pattern has been written for use in the home of the stroke patient. It is an attempt to describe to the stroke patient himself and *all* who care for him how best to help him to follow a way of life that will give him the maximum chance of a return to normal living. It is not an attempt to cut out the expert in rehabilitation; rather it is written so that the valuable work of the expert may be backed up in the home situation. Where expert domiciliary rehabilitation is given from the beginning by therapists and nurses, it will be rendered unproductive and improvement will not go forward as it should if lack of understanding leads to failure on the part of the home helper to undertaker 'positioning'. Where the family member — or whoever gives the round-the-clock attention — does not understand the patient's urgent need to **live in the recovery pattern**, the rehabilitation programme will almost certainly meet with failure. The same applies to the patient who is admitted to hospital and later returns home to continue with home rehabilitation.

There is no short cut to recovery. It is still necessary to think in terms of allowing recovery to go forward over months and, for obvious reasons, at least past — usually the greater part — of the long, slow fight to return to reasonable living takes place at home.

This book sets out to bring understanding to *all* who undertake the home care of a stroke patient, whatever their capacity, and, where possible, to bring understanding to the patient himself. He is the one who must live in this pattern.

A special effort has been made to point out the need for early and intensive treatment and, in particular, the vital need to maintain round-the-clock 'positioning'. Many hours are spent resting and sleeping in **the pattern**. Thus, intensive treatment does not mean excessive hard exercise. Early neglect can later lead to failure.

For the sake of clarity, throughout the text, the patient is referred to as 'he' and the therapist, nurse or helper as 'she'. In many places the reader is addressed directly as 'you', the assumption being that 'you', the reader, are the person most concerned with helping the stroke patient to help himself.

This new edition includes an update in the use of pressure splints without which it is not easy to offer progressive treatment. It is hoped that you, the reader, will find these splints helpful and that you may find in pressure splint techniques the answer to many of the patient's rehabilitation problems.

Edinburgh, 1987   M.J.

Contents

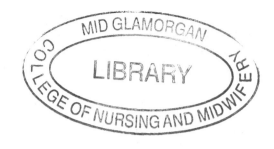

1.	A necessary introduction	1
2.	Rehabilitation	9
3.	Positioning	23
4.	Speech therapy *Sandra Jackson Anderson LCST*	65
5.	Progress through exercise	79
6.	Arm rehabilitation: extra help for the arm	144
7.	Case histories	180
	Glossary	213
	Appendix — some useful addresses	215
	Suggested further reading	216
	Index	217

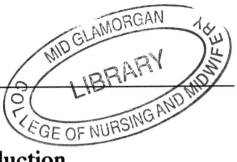
1

A necessary introduction

What is a stroke?

Damage to part of the brain will result if the blood supply to that part is interrupted and the sudden damage this causes gives the symptoms known as stroke. Other names are frequently used, such as shock, apoplexy, seizure, spasm, cerebrovascular accident (C.V.A.), cerebral thrombosis, but in recent years the word stroke has come to be more commonly used and is easier to understand. Stroke denotes the suddenness of onset and represents one of the worst features the patient has to contend with, namely the devastating shock he suffers when he realises that, in one unexpected moment and without prior warning, he has been denied the functional use of one half of his body; the half of the body on the opposite side to the site of brain damage. This is because nerve fibres leaving the brain cross to control the opposite side. Controlled movement is missing and his limbs refuse to obey him. Little wonder if he is depressed, irritable, even aggressive, because he is thoroughly frightened and quite helpless to attend to his own needs or to cope with the normal demands of daily living. Worse still, he may not be able to speak, or to make himself understood, though (except in a small minority of cases) he will understand all that is said to him. For all these reasons it is urgently necessary to establish hopeful and understanding communication with him as quickly as possible — be it only by mime.

Rehabilitation must begin immediately for many reasons, one being to show the patient physical improvement in his affected limbs so as to establish a beginning in self-care in the early dark days. Self-care will be the most important means used to lift his depression and to set him going on the road to recovery. Recovery, and finding a way back to normal living, will be very much in his own hands and the purpose of this book is to show his family and friends and all those who come into contact with him how best to help him to help himself. It is important not to make promises that cannot be kept and yet it is essential to approach him with cheerful optimism. Without hope the end result of recovery will be second best because a large part of success depends on the patient's own approach to rehabilitation. As

1

the purpose of this book is to throw light and understanding on a subject which is all too often misunderstood and badly handled perhaps this is the place where simple definitions ought to be given. Rehabilitation, then, means a planned programme in which the convalescent or disabled person progresses towards, or maintains, the maximum degree of physical and psychological independence of which he is capable. In the case of the stroke patient it is urgently necessary for rehabilitation to begin immediately after the onset of the disability.

What is the cause of a stroke?

A stroke is caused by bleeding into the brain from a ruptured blood vessel, or by blockage caused by thickening in an artery which supplies blood to the brain, or by a clot of blood which may have formed in the heart (or in an artery) and then broken away from its source to travel towards the brain. In the first case, the bleeding causes the damage. Bleeding inside the brain means that the ruptured blood vessel allows blood to flow into the brain cells, causing damage, and this is called a *cerebral haemorrhage.* In the second case, the moving clot is called an embolus and the stroke occurs when the embolus lodges in a position where it effectively cuts off blood supply to a part of the brain. Blockage of blood supply which thus may occur by gradual thickening of a vital artery wall, or by a travelling clot or embolus, is called a *cerebral thrombosis.* Whatever the cause, the end result occurs with dramatic suddenness and with devastating effects on the physical ability and emotional state of the patient.

Many people want to know what causes the haemorrhage or the thrombosis and this is not easy to say. The causes of stroke are not even clearly understood by the medical profession. Artery walls may become thickened and impregnated with lime salts, leading to narrowing and the tendency to burst. This may happen anywhere in the body but, because the brain is such a very complicated network of fibre tissues and nerve cells forming a very complicated computer all enclosed in the protective box which is the skull, there is no room for the expansion of the inflamed area produced by cerebral haemorrhage and the tight compression that results on such an intricate and delicate structure will lead to damage and to death of the cells most closely involved. Secondly (where the blood supply is cut off by cerebral thrombosis), without a blood supply there is no supply of oxygen, and no supply of oxygen to a cell results in the death of the cell. Probably the chief predisposing cause of stroke is high blood pressure (hypertension) and, because people with high blood pressure are more likely to have a stroke than those with normal blood pressure, doctors usually consider it well worthwhile to treat the condition. Also smoking is now known to carry many health hazards and very many doctors have themselves given up smoking.

Because a patient has had a stroke it does not follow that he can expect a second, or that he will ever have another. The chances of a second stroke will be greatly reduced if he follows his doctor's advice with care. In other words, if possible, the predisposing causes ought to be removed or treated. For example, anti-hypertensive drugs may be prescribed, smoking not allowed, animal fats reduced from the diet, blood disorders dealt with, diabetes kept under control, severe dehydration not permitted and, in some cases after cerebral embolus, anticoagulants may be ordered.

What are the symptoms of stroke?

The symptoms are many and varied. Immediately after onset the patient may be unconscious and this may last for hours, or even days. If it lasts for many days the outlook is generally not good. On the other hand the patient may be unconscious for a very short time or he may not lose consciousness at all. If he is conscious, or as soon as he regains consciousness, he will be upset, confused, bewildered and frightened and he may not be able to use an arm, or a leg, or both, or the whole of one side of his body — the side opposite to the injured area of his brain. He may not have full and normal feeling on one side of his body (usually the left), he may have visual difficulty, or he may not be able to speak (usually if he has right-sided weakness). He may also be incontinent. All this will be a direct result of the brain damage caused by the stroke. This is because nerve fibres from the brain pass down to cross to the opposite side of the spinal cord and spread out to supply the nerves and muscles which the brain controls. The fibres which come from the part of the brain that has been hit by the stroke then fail to control the parts these fibres supply. Also, when the sensory area of the brain is hit the supply fibres cannot send back to the brain the necessary messages of feeling — feeling, for example, which allows the brain to know the position a limb holds in relation to the rest of the body. The result is movement failure or paralysis.

It is necessary to understand that the smallest haemorrhage or the blockage of one small artery can effectively put an end to the control of the part of the body affected by the area hit. In other words, the muscles can no longer receive messages from the brain nor can those muscles send messages of feeling to the brain. As all controlled movements are a direct result of sensory messages it will be readily understood why the stroke patient is in deep trouble in the early dark days of disability.

Areas that may be affected

Figure 1 shows a diagram of the brain with its various areas. These are four in number, *motor, sensory, visual* and *auditory* and are each surrounded by the large areas which are associated with interpretation of *movement, feeling, seeing* and *hearing*. Each of the large areas is known as a lobe and each has a name — the *frontal, parietal, occipital* and *temporal* lobes. The need for this

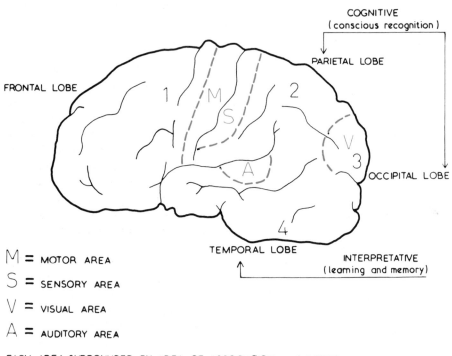

M = MOTOR AREA

S = SENSORY AREA

V = VISUAL AREA

A = AUDITORY AREA

EACH AREA SURROUNDED BY AREA OF ASSOCIATION = 4 LOBES

1 = FRONTAL LOBE (MOTOR)

2 = PARIETAL LOBE (SENSORY)

3 = OCCIPITAL LOBE (VISUAL)

4 = TEMPORAL LOBE (AUDITORY)

Fig. 1 Diagram of the four lobes of the brain

vast area of brain in man (and therefore the difficulties a patient may have after a stroke has reduced the efficiency of any area) may be better understood by giving a simple example. Suppose you put your hand into your pocket, find a fifty pence piece there and take hold of it with your thumb and two fingers. By feeling it, the sensory area of your brain (parietal lobe) recognises the shape of the coin and together parietal and occipital lobes allow *conscious recognition* to interpret the shape of the coin as that of a fifty pence piece. As you look at it, and going a step further, temporal lobe brings in *learning and memory* from past events which have been stored up and so the coin represents its value in terms of the goods it can buy. To me, if I withdrew the coin from my white coat pocket, it would most likely instantly represent my meal ticket for my daily hospital canteen lunch. Or again supposing I thrust my hand into my pocket and my fingers closed round another object I might find there. By feeling it the sensory area of my brain recognises the shape of a pencil. As I withdraw it from my pocket, the parietal and occipital lobes of my brain allow conscious recognition to interpret the shape as that of my favourite drawing pencil, a short and well-used treasure. I see that the point is blunt. Again going a step further, the temporal lobe of my brain brings in learning and memory from past events and so the pencil represents its value in terms of the many pictures it has produced, its life's expectancy, the need to sharpen the point, the cost of a new pencil and so on.

If brain damage is such that it prevents recognition of former familiar objects it follows that these objects cannot be related to present needs. To give an example of the difficulty that may face a stroke patient, it may be found that he cannot dress himself. His controlled movement, or motor power, may be intact but he does not recognise his clothes nor has he any idea what to do with them. He will have to start the relearning process of dressing and the patience and loving care with which this is attempted by his helper will have to equal the patience and care she would give to a tiny infant. She can expect the task of relearning to take many months. The patient must never be bullied, shouted at and roughly told that of course he can dress himself. Thus, where recognition is denied in the visual area, it must be clearly obvious that the patient will need very special help. That such a difficulty is present may be fairly easily picked up by a few simple assessment tests which a good remedial therapist may carry out either in hospital or in the patient's room. Assessment tests may be used to pick out difficulties in all areas and may need a combined team of physiotherapist, occupational therapist and speech therapist.

Areas that may be affected (pinpointing difficulties)

1. *Muscles*. There may be paralysis of one side of the body which is called hemiplegia. There may be slight loss of strength in one arm and one leg and this is called hemiparesis. There may be facial weakness on the same side which leads to dribbling from the weak side of the mouth and there

may be difficulty in chewing and swallowing. There may be speech difficulty (see below).

2. *Feeling*. There may be loss of feeling on the affected side of the body, or loss of awareness, which may mean that the patient will perhaps not recognise the affected half of his own body, its position in space or its relation to the rest of his body. As shown above, he may not be able to recognise objects and texture by touch and, worse still, he may not recognise objects by sight or have the remotest idea of their purpose or what to do with them. It should be understood that this is not blindness but a difficulty in perception. For example he might sit with a bowl of soup in front of him and make no effort to use the spoon because of damage to the association areas of conscious recognition and interpretation. He does not recognise the spoon or its use.

3. *Sight*. There may be difficulty in seeing out of one half of each eye; if the left half of the body is affected the patient may not see out of the left half of both eyes. This is blindness. The doctor will call it hemianopia.

4. *Speech*. As stated above, the patient may have lost the ability to speak — or to speak clearly — because the muscles involved in speech are not functioning properly. This is a difficulty with forming words and not a difficulty with language and is called dysarthria. The patient will have no difficulty in understanding the spoken word and he can usually write. On the other hand, he may have difficulty in finding words, a disorder of language which is called dysphasia. Dysphasia may simply involve the patient's output of words, but, in a small percentage of cases, it may include input — or recognition and interpretation of the spoken word. More usually the patient's comprehension has remained intact. Because speech and language problems may present in many and varied ways and can only be properly assessed and understood by the specialist, it is urgently necessary in this field to seek the advice of a qualified speech therapist. It ought to be noted that it may not even be obvious to the lay person that there is difficulty in this field when there may be difficulty and it may be causing the patient real distress. Home treatment by the attentive family and friends may be able to do much to help some speech and language problems *but* active harm may be done by lack of understanding of the problem presented in any one case and, consequently, by making a wrong and harmful approach. It ought to be accepted that home treatment for speech and language disorders should only be given under the careful guidance of a qualified speech therapist.

5. *Emotion*. Emotion might have been included under the heading, *feeling*, but is given a separate heading here because it involves feeling in the mind as distinct from feeling by touch. Nevertheless, emotion, a moving of the feelings or agitation of mind, is part of cognition. By dictionary definition, cognition means awareness, one of the three aspects of mind, the others being affection (feeling or emotion) and conation (willing or desiring). They work as a whole but any one may dominate any

mental process. In stroke care we must consider emotional upset because it is an area which may be very seriously disturbed. The patient may weep easily and find it hard to get a grip of himself. A former emotionally stable and strong character may become temperamental, highly excitable, over-sensitive, impatient, changeable and deeply unhappy. Emotional upset and depression are frequently present, particularly in the early grim days after the sudden onset of a stroke with its resulting disability.

A cheerful approach to the patient offering correct methods of rehabilitation can go a long way towards reducing emotional distress. Each step forward in recovery will lead away from the frustration and depression that may be brought on by the patient's feeling of helpless inadequacy because he has suddenly had to undergo the humiliating experience of becoming dependent on the help of others. It would be surprising if a body that is suddenly found to be out of control and that will not respond to former normal demands retained a quiet and cheerful spirit.

By the same token, where willing and desiring are affected, the patient may show disinterest in his condition or his progress in rehabilitation. Indeed, progress will be very slow if it occurs at all. Rehabilitation may be offered, he may be shown what he must do to help himself, but the helper's task will be doubly difficult where this area is affected by his stroke. A way *must* be found to stimulate his interest. In modern jargon, disinterest will certainly be a contributing factor to poor motivation! But, again, it is frequently found that to show a patient a degree (however small) of physical improvement in his condition is to make the first positive step towards lifting his mood of disinterested apathy. This is what rehabilitation is all about.

6. *Incontinence and constipation*. Initially bladder control may be poor or missing but this usually adjusts fairly quickly. Constipation may be a quite serious problem, probably because of loss of tone in the gut in the early days. The patient may appear to be troubled by diarrhoea but this may very well be a leaking past a blockage because of constipation difficulty high up in the colon. The doctor's help ought to be sought if there is any marked change in pre-stroke habits in this area.

7. *Sex life*. It is important for the patient to understand, as he gets better and resumes normal living, that there is no reason why he should not resume a former normal married relationship. An understanding partner will help in this area and he himself must be reassured (if necessary by his doctor). There is no medical reason for abandoning a former way of life. Any doubts or difficulties whatsoever in this area ought to be discussed with the doctor.

Initial care of the stroke patient

The first step in the care of a stroke patient will be in the hands of the family doctor. Immediately after the stroke an urgent call must be sent out for the attention of the family doctor. There must be no delay.

While waiting for the doctor to arrive the patient should be kept warm. If he is unconscious he ought to be rolled over on to his front with his head turned sideways so that his airway is clear for freedom in breathing and his tongue must stay forward in his mouth making sure he does not choke. When the doctor arrives the patient's immediate future will be decided by him. The doctor has to choose between home or hospital care and he knows best which choice to make. Some families may resist the suggestion of admission to hospital but the doctor will assess all the circumstances and he is the only one in a position to know what must be done in his patient's best interest. Here, previous knowledge of the family will help him and he will also consider his patient's needs from every angle. Where he considers special nursing is necessary, where diagnostic facilities are needed, where rehabilitation services are inadequate in the community, or where he knows the household would break down under the strain of immediate home care he will advise hospital admission. In a few cases he may call in a hospital consultant physician to help make the decision. If the patient is to be nursed at home, other services (e.g. health visitors, district nurses, domiciliary physiotherapists, social workers and the home help service) may have to become involved and the home help service may be the make or break point when the decision is made. Services are scarce but if the level of rehabilitation offered at home could be equal to hospital care it would be of tremendous value. At the time of writing, in a small minority of cases the level of home care is equal to, or superior to, hospital care. One of the aims of this book is to help weight the balance in favour of home-care — if not immediately after the stroke at least as continuing care after discharge. Recovery must continue and sound methods of rehabilitation must be offered.

Frequently, an initial short period of hospital care is essential but the patient will be sent home as soon as possible and he will almost certainly still be in need of skilled rehabilitation if he is not to remain severely disabled. Whatever the decision, rehabilitation should begin at once and the assistance of caring relatives is of supreme importance. If the patient must go to hospital it is to be hoped the relatives will be encouraged by the hospital to join rehabilitation sessions and to learn what it is all about so that they are well qualified to take over correct handling when their family member returns home. The help of a domiciliary physiotherapist may be needed but in many cases the caring family member ought to be ready to take over with very little supervision.

2

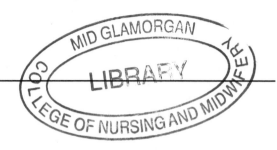

Rehabilitation

What is it all about?

Rehabilitation consists of a planned programme in which the convalescent or disabled person progresses towards, or maintains, the maximum degree of physical and psychological independence of which he is capable. To learn and to understand what rehabilitation of the stroke patient is all about it is necessary to understand what has happened to the patient in terms of the physical disability he may have to face. To understand the physical disability of a stroke and how best to help the patient, it is urgently necessary to understand a few simple facts about movement and the normal controlled movement the healthy human being takes very much for granted. He is not born with controlled movement: he is born with what is called primitive reflex movement. He spends the first months of his life developing motor control. He works through primitive reflex happenings until they become part of controlled posture and voluntary movement. In other words he progresses through the stages of reflex movement to postural control to voluntary movement to learned skills. He is walking upright, he has developed precision movements and learns skilled movements which are intended to last him a lifetime. The basic reflexes which he used as foundation bricks on which to build his controlled movement are still with him but they are integrated into postural control. Some of them — those that support him against gravity — are dominant, or stronger, than others but this does not matter, his brain is in control and he is his own man. Sadly, after a stroke, his brain is no longer in control and he is no longer his own man. This devastating truth hits him out of the blue and this is the first grim fact he must attempt to face. He is called on to come to terms with the knowledge that he is in many respects quite helpless, one half of his body will no longer obey him, balance is missing, normal movement on his affected side is no longer possible and he is in some respects as dependent on the help of others as a newborn child. He cannot even take himself to the privacy of the lavatory, but must be taken and helped like a small child. He feels degraded, in many ways much less than half a man; he is dejected, dispirited, and often deeply troubled. Usually his spirits sink to a very low ebb. It is urgently necessary to offer him the right kind of help. Before any helper is in a position to offer the support that is so urgently needed, he or she must understand the normal development patterns that lead to normal motor control.

Figure 2 shows some of the positions and movement patterns adopted by the infant as he passes through the various stages of motor development. In the process of development, controlled movement of the neck and shoulders comes before elbow and finally hand control; controlled movement of the trunk and hip before the knee and foot. This illustration may also be used to demonstrate the importance weight-bearing has on the development of controlled movement. The baby must prop on his forearms and progress to standing on his knees *and on his hands* in the normal crawling patterns he adopts while he passes through the various stages of development. Without this weight-bearing his progress would not move forward and he would not reach his goal, i.e. controlled posture and co-ordinated movement.

Put another way, development is from head to foot, or, in the simple development pattern seen in the infant, the primitive reflexes lead from lips and tongue, to eye muscles, to neck, shoulder, arms, hands, fingers, trunk, legs, feet, the primitive responses giving way to controlled movement and posture. Or, as we say, primitive movement becomes automatic and then deliberate or purposeful. The infant can control his arms and hands before his legs and feet. In the final stages of development of fully co-ordinated movement the hand and the foot take over and, instead of following the lead given by the shoulder and hip, they initiate movement and the hand in particular becomes the leader in co-ordinated, functional and skilled movement. Just think of the development patterns you watched in your own child, or a brother or sister, or a grandchild and you will remember the course it took. (An important note here for later reference: if the normal development patterns are interrupted by the exclusive use of a baby bouncer in which the child swings in upright suspension and bounces by an upward thrust on his feet in response to pressure on the forepart of his feet he will stimulate his extensor reflex to such an extent he will not be able to sit down).

But how does all this relate to the stroke patient? Why talk about the infant's development of controlled movement when considering the rehabilitation of the stroke patient? Firstly, let's consider Figure 3.

In Figure 3 we see a picture of the tiny baby who has no controlled movement. All his movements are primitive or reflex. For example, at this stage he may turn his head, moves his eyes, grasp with his fingers, kick his legs rapidly, or even appear to take a deliberate step if he is held upright with his feet touching a firm surface, but these are all responses to primitive reflex happenings and they are not purposeful controlled movements.

Where would he be without his sucking reflex? Because of his sucking reflex he can feed but he cannot stand up and go and get his own bottle.

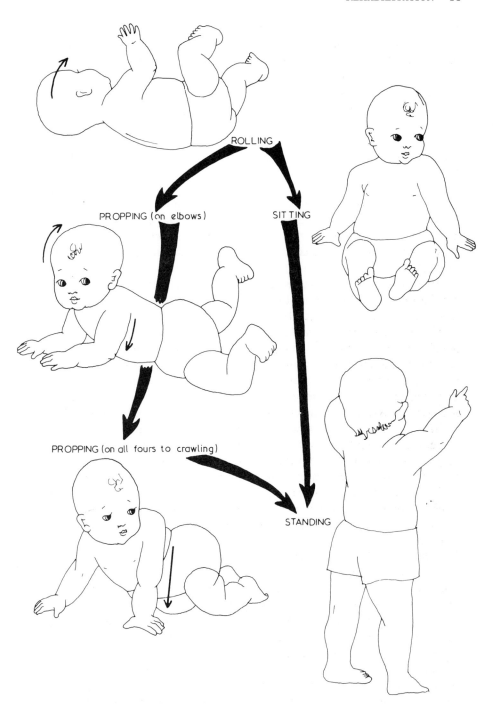

ROLLING

PROPPING (on elbows)

SITTING

PROPPING (on all fours to crawling)

STANDING

Fig. 2 Development of controlled movement in the infant

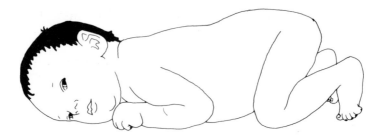

Fig. 3 The human infant

Sensory stimulation round the mouth leads to a response which sets off a whole chain of reflex happenings from lips and tongue, to eye muscles, to mouth and so on as described above. His whole programme of development is dependent on these chain reactions. Rotation of his neck with flexion of his trunk to the same side leads to arm flexion. Tilting his head backwards makes him stetch out, or extend, his arms and bend, or flex, his hips and knees. Or lifting his head backwards when he is lying on his face makes him push on his forearms and hands and extend his upper spine. Or, if he lies on his tummy and lifts his head and turns it, he pushes more strongly on the arm towards which he turns and this leads to rolling over on to his back. He is equipped at birth with what we call postural and righting reflexes and these are quite simply the reflexes that lead him eventually to hold his head upright in space and to stand upright against gravity. When he holds his head upright in space his body follows. When he has achieved this we say his primitive postural reflexes have integrated into controlled posture and controlled movement follows. His brain is in command because he has worked right up through the different levels of reflex activity (from below upwards the levels are spinal, tonic, basal and so to the cerebral cortex) and the higher centres of the brain have established control.

So, as shown in Figure 2, head lifting and turning leads to rolling, rolling to propping, propping to crawling, and crawling to standing. Also rolling leads to sitting and sitting to standing. Both of these advancing patterns are used but some babies use one more than the other. All through the early days of growth and development, the baby's progress moves forwards as a result of the constant repetition of movements in response to built-in reflex action. But why should he lift and rotate his head in the first place? As a response to sensory stimulation, touch, vision and hearing creating the demand that gains the response. All movement is a response to sensory stimulation. As describe above, without stimulation of sensation round the mouth the primitive sucking reflex would not follow. Sensory development and movement development go forward together until developmental growth is complete.

Thus, as just suggested, at birth the baby's development towards controlled movement has reached primitive reflex level with all his movements occurring as a result of reflex action. But what of his sensory development?

Here a simple review of our understanding of **sensory** development helps our understanding of the planned development of a worthwhile stroke rehabilitation programme. Before birth, as the fetus grows, the **major inputs** to the developing nervous system are the various sensations of *touch, movement and pressure.* The fetus is surrounded by fluid and enclosed in the uterus so that the entire skin surface is subjected to altering pressures. As the mother moves and alters her posture, pressures on the fetus alter. As she walks the developing baby rocks in the uterus. There is also the rhythmic increase and decrease in pressures that corresponds with the mother's respiration rate. Overall pressures will increase as the baby grows.

These are the sensations that signal safety and comfort so no wonder the newborn baby cries. Some zoologists even describe it as a scream of terror. During the last 3 months of pregnancy it is also known that the fetus can hear; this means that the mother's heart-beat is the first sound imprinted on the developing brain. The mother who cradles the baby in her arms, who walks up and down rocking the baby and holding it close with its head held where it will hear her heart-beat, is instinctively mimicking the 'embrace' of the uterus in these efforts to comfort and reassure the baby.

To sum up, at birth movement has reached primitive reflex level and, in the following months, as movement development progresses up through the reflex levels — **spinal, tonic, basal** — to reach **cortical** control and learned skills (or to establish the normal postural reflex mechanism where the brain is in command and normal movement is established) *at the same time* **sensory** *development continues.* It would seem then that in the light of what has been said about the prenatal influences of **touch, movement** and **pressure** on the developing fetus, it would make sense to use pressures, and altering pressures, when setting out to restore *normal sensation and normal movement* in the stroke patient. And that is what is done.

Figure 4 shows the stages an average baby follows to establish crawling and it should be remembered, in these developmental patterns his whole body is constantly subjected to altering weight-bearing pressures. Added methods for increasing the necessary programme to give the stroke patient altering pressures will be presented later in the text.

After birth the baby turns his head to the side, usually towards the window which is the source of light. His limbs curl up in flexion.

At the end of the first month he can lift his head and hold it up for about three seconds.

At the end of the second month he can usually hold his head up for about ten seconds.

By the end of the fifth month he may attempt to roll and he also 'swims' when he lies on his tummy by supporting himself and lifting his head, chest and arms.

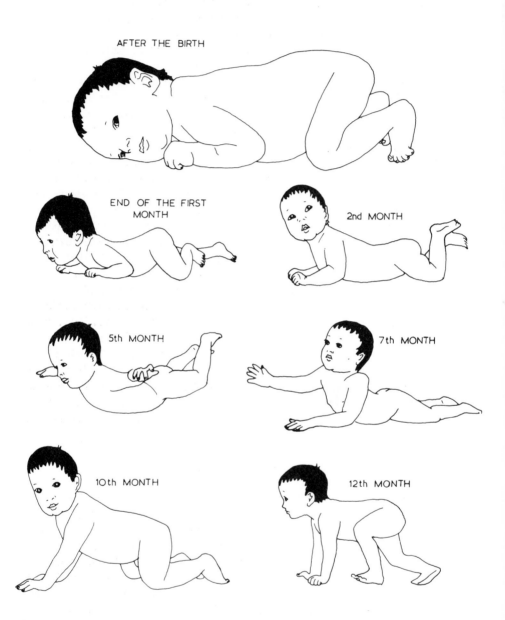

Fig. 4 Stages of the infant's motor development

By the seventh month he can reach for something in front of him while lying on his tummy and supporting himself on the other arm.

By the tenth month, after learning to pull himself along with his arms, he now starts crawling on hands and knees.

By the eleventh and twelfth months he starts getting up on to his feet. He is well on the way to establishing full control.

So, what have Figures 2, 3 and 4 to do with the stroke patient? Quite simply they are presented as an aid to understanding the physical disability that faces the stroke patient and therefore as the key that opens the door leading to recovery. *We must relate the infant's pattern of motor development to our stroke patient.* Depending on the severity of onset, half of his body has become, at a stroke and with devastating suddenness, akin to that of a newborn infant. He is left with primitive reflex movement; voluntary controlled movement is out of his reach because brain damage has interfered with the normal postural reflex mechanism he spent so many months developing at the beginning of his life. In the words of the physiotherapist, the primitive reflexes are no longer integrated into controlled movement. The stronger, or dominant, reflexes will gain the upper hand and over a period of weeks or months will produce the spastic, twisted body that many of us have seen in the past and which is instantly recognised as stroke disability. Add to this the fact that the patient will have muscle weakness because the motor pathways to the affected muscles have been interrupted and things may be further complicated by sensory loss. It has already been shown that all movement is a response to sensory stimulation. Is it any wonder he is in trouble? To a greater or lesser degree, according to the severity of the stroke, one half of his body is out of control. There is no time to lose. It is urgently necessary to offer him help; *but* it must be the right kind of help, the wrong kind will multiply his difficulties and he will never be his own man again.

The right kind of help

What is the right kind of help? The doctor makes the initial decisions about the best and right way to care for his patient and he will continue for some time (whether he be the family doctor or his hospital colleague) to take over all responsibility for looking after his patient's welfare, but rehabilitation is the most important part of stroke treatment. The doctor offers the required medication and hands over rehabilitation to those who care for his patient. If the patient is admitted to hospital, nurses and therapists undertake initial rehabilitation and then, if possible, they will later hand over to the family; or the patient may stay at home and the family and community services will help from the beginning. So the right kind of help consists of good rehabilitation, again emphasising that to rehabilitate means to restore, or to bring back into good condition. How do we set about restoring the stroke patient? We must offer him the exercise routines that will give him the best possible chance of recovery. But the family member will only be able to offer the right and the best rehabilitation if he or she understands the reasoning behind the method used. That is what this book is all about.

What are the exercise routines? From what has already been said the answer to this question might seem obvious. Simply teach the patient to follow the exercise patterns as shown in Figures 2 and 4; that is, copy the routines the infant uses in his early months to gain co-ordinated and controlled posture and movement? This is exactly what must be done. Start with rolling and where the patient has the added complication of problems of speech, language, or perception we will hope that these may resolve as treatment progresses. After all, the baby does not talk before he walks! In any case, where there is any speech or language difficulty we must ask for the help of the speech therapist. She may also give helpful advice about dealing with perceptual problems and her assessment, which is highly specialised, is very valuable.

But there are two other complications, or barriers to the rehabilitation of controlled movement. They have so far been touched on very briefly but they *must* be taken into account. They are the biggest hurdles blocking the way to physical recovery and the patient must have help to get over them. They are:

1. Developing spasticity
2. Possible sensory loss which may be minimal or very severe

We are therefore considering three difficulties when we set out to offer the stroke patient the right kind of help. It might be helpful to make a list of them here:

1. In the beginning we must consider the patient's affected side to be as helpless as a newborn infant (Fig. 3). Because of this we cannot expect him to have full voluntary and controlled movement on his affected side and he will have lost balance.

2. However floppy his limbs may be immediately after the onset of the stroke *spasticity will develop*. If this is allowed to happen it will put an end to rehabilitation and the whole exercise programme will fail.

3. He may have some degree of sensory loss and sensory failure leads to movement failure because all controlled movements are a direct response to sensory messages.

Having reached the decision that it is necessary to relate the infant's patterns of motor development to the stroke patient, does this mean that developing spasticity and sensory loss may put an end to all hope of successfully carrying through the planned programme of rehabilitation? The answer to this question must be *yes*, spasticity and sensory loss may very well put an end to any progress the patient might make and reduce a reasonable hope of recovery to dismal failure *unless special measures are taken*. Spasticity and/or sensory loss may very well bring the planned programme of rehabilitation to an abrupt halt almost before it has begun.

For example, no stroke patient can learn to crawl on hands and knees if he develops a tightly fisted hand with a stiff flexed wrist. And if the patient has lost all feeling of joint and muscle sense so that he has no idea of a limb's position in space, how can he begin to move it and follow the vital rolling, crawling and balancing routines? In this last case it will be found that developing spasticity is less of a problem but the sensory loss is an even bigger hurdle in the way of success. *But* it is essential to embark on the necessary planned programme of rehabilitation exercises and to carry them through to a successful conclusion. The right kind of help is most urgently needed if the development of spasticity is to be prevented and sensory loss overcome. Again, understanding will lead to the right kind of help because *there is a way round these difficulties.* This leads to more questions to which answers must be found.

Why spasticity?

The clue to the answer to this vexed question has already been given. To quote: 'Some reflexes — those that support man against gravity — are dominant, or stronger, than others but this does not matter, his brain is in control and he is his own man.' With the stroke patient this is no longer true. The side affected by the stroke is no longer fully commanded by the brain, the captain of the ship is missing and the dominant or stronger reflexes take over from the weaker and produce the patterns of spasticity, or the typical spasticity pattern of the stroke patient. This affects the anti-gravity muscle groups that extend the body into the upright position against gravity and those that are used in the arms to lift weight against gravity.

Figure 5 represents a gibbon hanging by his left hand and thrusting upward with his right foot. This illustration is used because it gives a very clear picture of anti-gravity muscles, particularly the anti-gravity muscles of the arm. Failure to rehabilitate the arm of the stroke patient frequently occurs because this arm pattern is not understood and the resulting residual problem of the stroke arm makes normal living impossible. Gibbons live high in trees where they travel by swinging by their arms fully using the anti-gravity muscles of the arms. They are the most agile of mammals, indeed their agility is quite incredible. They also make apparently effortless leaps of 30 feet or more and their reflexes match their agility. This means that the gibbon makes a very good subject to use as an illustration of dominant reflexes. Man's dominant reflexes follow exactly the same pattern but a photograph of man does not show this nearly as clearly as a photograph of the gibbon. Study Figure 5 and it will be seen that the gibbon is using his anti-gravity muscles of his left arm and his right leg. With his arm he is hanging by one hand with his shoulder rolled or turned *inwards* — or in internal rotation — and he is just beginning to pull himself upwards by flexing his elbow while he assists the movement by thrusting upward on his right leg, extending the knee. Note that the hip is turned *outwards* — or in

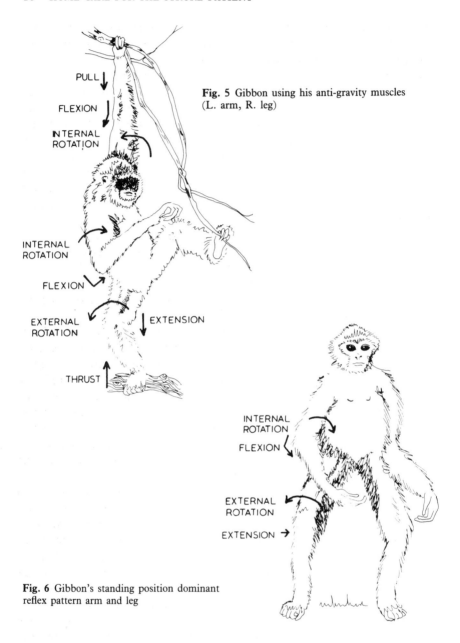

PULL

FLEXION

INTERNAL
ROTATION

Fig. 5 Gibbon using his anti-gravity muscles
(L. arm, R. leg)

INTERNAL
ROTATION

FLEXION

EXTERNAL
ROTATION   EXTENSION

THRUST

INTERNAL
ROTATION

FLEXION

EXTERNAL
ROTATION

EXTENSION

Fig. 6 Gibbon's standing position dominant
reflex pattern arm and leg

external rotation. Also note that the right arm shows the resting position,
dominant reflexes maintaining a pull downwards and backwards on the
shoulder with marked internal rotation of the shoulder while the elbow,
wrist and fingers go into marked flexion. This is a perfect picture of the
spasticity pattern the arm will adopt in the stroke patient. In the illustration

the left leg is not at rest, the gibbon is holding a branch with his toes but it is clearly seen by the position of his right leg which has almost reached full upward thrust, the dominant (therefore spasticity) pattern would be full extension on a hip that is rolled outwards in full external rotation.

Figure 6 shows the gibbon's standing position — again showing the dominant reflex patterns for both the arm and the leg very clearly. It should be said that gibbons are also very agile on the ground and, because their reflexes match their incredible agility, they make the perfect animal on which to study the dominant anti-gravity reflexes. Apart from man, they are the only apes that habitually walk upright on their hindlegs. When walking on the ground or along a branch they hold their arms out to help in balancing but again, as in Figure 6, the arms turn inwards with forearm flexion — the dominant pattern. Relate all this to man and the spasticity pattern of the stroke patient ought to be easily understood. Man uses his legs in a similar way to the gibbon although he no longer swings through the trees by his arms. However he still has a very strong group of shoulder muscles which give the original *very strong downward pull into internal rotation* and all heavy lifting and carrying is done by bracing these muscles and flexing his forearms, just as seen in the gibbon.

In the early days after a stroke the patient's limbs on his affected side may be weak, floppy and quite useless but, even at this stage, it is most important to take precautions against the slow, insidious onset of creeping spasticity which, once it becomes fully established (usually within 18 months), will lock the affected limbs into a non-functional, useless and painful pattern as described above which will successfully put an end to all worthwhile rehabilitation. The trouble is that much of the help and support offered by all those who care for the stroke victim may be a contributing factor to the build up of spasticity. Why this should happen should become clear as the reader studies this book.

Rehabilitation is the most important part of stroke treatment *but* a successful outcome can only be expected if this build-up of spasticity is prevented. *And it can be prevented.* But it can only be prevented if all those who have any dealings whatsoever with the patient adopt the correct measures to hold it in check while recovery takes place. This careful restraining of the stronger or dominant reflexes must continue until recovery has reached a stage where voluntary controlled movement takes over. Then the captain of the ship (the brain) once more takes command. At home, the family will play the most important part in this prevention of developing spasticity and it is most helpful where possible to teach the patient to take over the care of his own limbs. Help that is offered will not be effective and the battle against developing spasticity will not be won if the problem is not understood. So it is useless to discuss the patient's rehabilitation at home where the family is involved unless the caring family member is very carefully taught how to deal with the problem of spasticity. Again, this is what this book is all about.

How can spasticity be prevented?

The patient must be placed in, nursed in, handled in and taught to use the anti-spasticity positions and patterns twenty-four hours a day. Even the furniture he uses must be placed correctly. This is not as complicated as it may sound. It is really quite simple. Initially he must be nursed, handled and placed in the opposite pattern to the spasticity pattern at all times and then he is taught and helped to maintain this pattern round the clock. An adequate number of pillows will be essential for use at night while the patient sleeps. This diligent care of the patient's limbs that is so necessary to prevent developing spasticity is called positioning. For the stroke patient positioning must become a way of life while recovery is actively encouraged and allowed to happen. This means the patient is taught to live in the recovery pattern at all times.

Before going on to discuss the methods used to encourage recovery it is necessary to understand exactly what is meant by positioning in the recovery pattern. Again this is not a complicated thing to learn. It simply means positioning the patient in the opposite pattern to the pattern of spasticity. It may be called the recovery pattern, or the anti-spasticity pattern, but it is directly opposed to the spasticity pattern and it is the position which allows the maximum recovery to take place. To give a single and very important example, spasticity (because of the dominant anti-gravity pattern) turns the shoulder and arm into internal rotation so positioning is used to counter this by always maintaining the shoulder and arm in external rotation. Return to Figure 5 and think of the gibbon hoisting himself upward against gravity by pulling strongly on the upstretched arm which then flexes strongly on *an internally rotated shoulder*. As illustrated, he is also pushing strongly on an extended leg which is *externally rotated at the hip*. As already decided, both of these actions are against gravity and effectively show the anti-gravity muscles which are the same in man. We can forget the gibbon. He has served his purpose and given a very clear picture of anti-gravity muscles and therefore the developing patterns of spasticity we can expect to find in any stroke patient if no preventive measures are taken. Now *study Figures 7 and 8*. In Figure 7, the stick man represents the spasticity pattern on the red, or affected, side while Figure 8 shows the anti-spasticity or recovery pattern which is directly opposed to the pattern in Figure 7. In other words, Figure 8 shows the position that must be remembered, maintained and used all through rehabilitation. Again it must be stressed that this is not a complicated thing to learn and once it is mastered it will be seen how relatively easily it may be maintained in all situations. Better still, it is often fairly quickly understood and mastered by the patient himself provided careful teaching is given. Begin by thinking in terms of the two most important joints, the shoulder and the hip. To keep within the recovery pattern the shoulder must not be allowed to turn inwards and the hip must not be allowed to turn outwards. This means that the upper

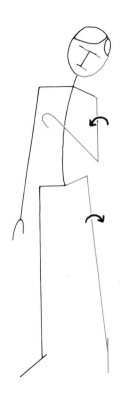

Drawing back of shoulder with depression and INTERNAL ROTATION.

Elbow bent.

Fingers bent and close together.

Drawing back of hip with EXTERNAL ROTATION of the leg.

Hip, knee and ankle straight with forefoot and toes pointing down.

Fig. 7 Spasticity pattern in red

Drawing forward of shoulder with EXTERNAL ROTATION.

Forearm straight.

Fingers straight and separated.

Drawing forward of the hip with INTERNAL ROTATION of the leg.

Hip, knee and ankle bent.

Fig. 8 Anti-spasticity or recovery pattern

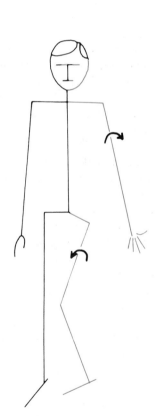

arm should be supported in a forward position with the *shoulder joint turned outwards* or in external rotation. To get this position right in the early days it is helpful to turn the palm of the hand forward with the thumb pointing away from the body. The upper thigh should also be supported in a forward position so that the knee is slightly flexed (or fully flexed to 90° when the patient is sitting in a chair) and *the hip joint turns inwards* or is in internal rotation. It is at once obvious that these two important joints follow opposite patterns — the shoulder must be kept in external rotation and the hip in internal rotation while both are supported in a forward position. Each of these patterns is the direct opposite of the spasticity pattern. If this is found by the reader to cause any confusion the diagrams that follow will help to establish this most important business of correct *positioning*. As rehabilitation is built round correct positioning for twenty-four hours of every day, in the hospital situation it is not something a therapist can undertake alone. It must be based on the patient's whole way of life. No therapist, single-handed and seeing a patient for a short time each day, can possibly prevent the development of spasticity. She can only show other people how it is done; she must hand over to the nurses (and the family) who are with the patient round the clock. This means that in the early days where hospital care is necessary the family ought to be involved. In any case sooner or later the family must be involved and sooner is much better than later. Improvement can be expected for many months and treatment must continue all through those months if the patient is to be given a reasonable hope of returning to normal living. More and more of this treatment is being done at home and, where this is possible, this is the ideal situation. Careful positioning and correct handling with a clear understanding of how to deal with the problem of spasticity will go a long way towards promoting recovery, and a patient will usually recover best in his own surroundings. Because the prevention of developing spasticity is such an important part of stroke rehabilitation, and therefore of recovery, it is proposed to go into *positioning* in detail so that the phrase *living in the pattern of recovery* is fully understood.

3

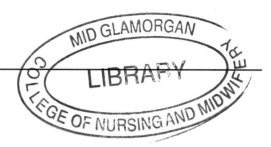

Positioning

Positioning of the patient's furniture

As already stated, the patient's correct positioning and handling must also include the correct positioning of his furniture so this seems an appropriate place to insert a diagram to this effect. In other words, get the furniture right from the beginning.

Figure 9 shows the correct positioning of the patient's immediate furniture for left-sided weakness. For right-sided weakness the table (or locker) and chair would be placed on the other side of the bed. When a commode is in use it should always be placed in the position which gives the patient the greatest chance of managing independently. As soon as he has learnt to get himself in and out of bed using the chair in the position as shown in Figure 9b, the commode ought to be placed in the chair's position for night use. For day use it ought to be removed altogether and brought to the bedside and correctly positioned only if it is needed. However, if the patient is to be left alone for an hour or two when he has passed through the initial stages of gaining independence, it ought to be placed as shown in Figure 9c so that he can transfer himself from chair to commode and back again. For his self-respect it ought to have a lid. If he is given the suggested cantilever table (Fig. 11) for use while he sits out of bed, when necessary he will be able to push it out of the way over the bed as shown in Figure 9c.

Figures 10 and 11 illustrate the type of furniture the patient ought to be given. The chair should have a broad base, solid forearm supports, a comfortably upright back and be virtually impossible to tip. It must also be the right height to allow him to sit comfortably with his hips, knees and ankles at right angles.

With the help of suitable furniture correctly positioned the patient is ready to begin rehabilitation, starting as in Figure 9a. The next thing is to get the patient's positioning right. As soon as this is established it will be seen why the bed, chair, tables, commode and even the television must occupy the places shown in the diagrams. Further points on furniture and positioning of furniture for the mobile patient will be given later.

23

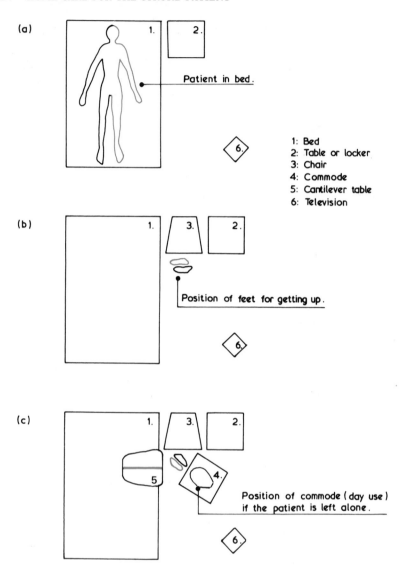

Fig. 9 Positioning of patient's furniture

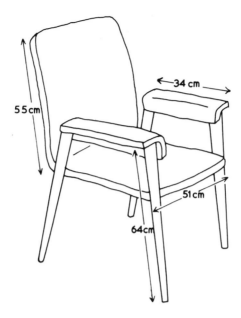

Fig. 10 Suitable chair

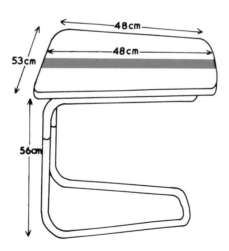

Fig. 11 Cantilever table

Positioning of the patient in bed plus bed exercises

As stated before, the first aim of all treatment is to prevent the development of spasticity. Incorrect positioning of the patient while he lies in bed, whether he be conscious or unconscious, will inevitably lead to the beginning of this unwanted build-up of spasticity. In the words of the physiotherapist it is very necessary to prevent the build-up of unwanted reflex action. This means that at all times nothing must be done which encourages unwanted reflex action or build-up of spasticity patterns. In the early days of treatment this means that at all times the patient's limbs must be placed away from the direction of pull of the patterns of spasticity. As already shown in Figures 7 and 8, the limbs must be placed not in the pattern of the strong anti-gravity muscles but in the pattern of the weaker opposing muscles — the *hip* and knee slightly bent with the leg *rolled inwards,* the *shoulder* lifted forwards and the arm *rolled outwards* with the elbow and wrist straight. If in any doubt about the position of the arm, remember to turn the palm of the hand forward so that it faces outward with the thumb pointing away from the body. It is also necessary to prevent shortening of the trunk on the affected side by not allowing the patient to lie bent to that side. This may tend to happen because of spasticity in the back muscles on the affected side. Sometimes it may not be possible to maintain the affected limbs in the complete anti-spasticity pattern the entire twenty-four hours of every day. In that case, part of the pattern must be maintained and, again, it is most helpful to the patient if the correct positioning of the hip and shoulder are given first priority.

If the following points are noted, full (or an acceptable degree of) corrective positioning will be maintained while the patient lies in bed. In other words, at all times the positioning of the patient and his furniture is undertaken in the ways suggested in this book in order to influence the distribution of his muscle tone. This corrective positioning is used *to inhibit the build-up of excessive anti-gravity tone.*

1. *Lying on the back,* as shown in Figure 12, is the position which must be used with the greatest care because this is the position which will most easily allow the unwanted spasticity to develop. This is because the head tends to press back into the pillow giving the unwanted extension of the spine, the arm tends to drop backwards with the shoulder in the unwanted pattern of internal rotation and the hip, knee and foot all readily adopt the forbidden pattern of extension as used against gravity in standing with the leg rolling into unwanted external rotation. Therefore, when lying on the back cannot be avoided, the head should be well supported, the affected shoulder also carefully supported by pillows so that it is lifted forward with the arm slightly raised and rolled outward with the elbow and wrist straight and the thumb pointing away from the body. At the same time, a pillow is placed under the hip to prevent the hip joint from dropping backward and rolling outward. Always remember that the hip and shoulder joints are

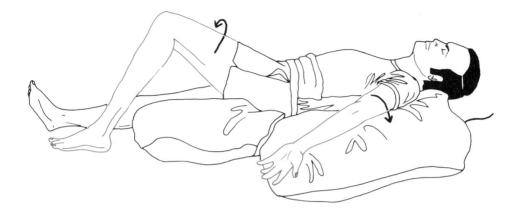

Fig. 12 Lying on the back

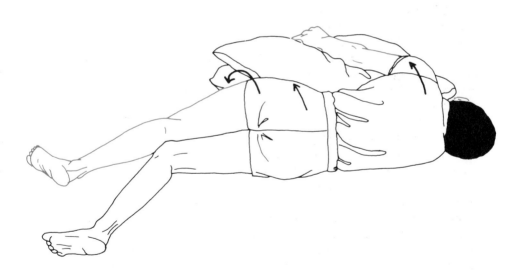

Fig. 13 Lying on the sound side

placed in opposite patterns, the hip is rolled inwards and the shoulder outwards. If in any doubt, again consult Figure 12 which gives a clear indication of the position which ought to be maintained when the patient lies on his back. The amount of knee bend may be as much or as little as the patient finds comfortable as long as it is bent and the leg is not allowed to roll outwards. Again there ought to be an adequate number of supporting pillows to maintain the position. Try and avoid hard pressure on the calf muscles. As illustrated in Figure 12, the patient has been carefully positioned. Additional supporting pillows will be required.

2. *Lying on the sound side*, as shown in Figure 13, is a good position provided the patient is fully on his side and the limbs on the affected side are carefully positioned. The affected shoulder is again brought foward and the arm is not allowed to roll inwards. This is quite simply achieved by placing the affected arm well forward across supporting pillows. The affected leg is also placed forward with only one supporting pillow so that the hip is allowed to roll inwards into internal rotation.

3. *Lying on the affected side*, as shown in Figure 14, will not build up spasticity and ought to be used some of the time (particularly where there is loss of feeling on the affected half of the body, a point which will be noted later). But it must be understood that this is the position which will be most uncomfortable for the patient and will do most damage to the affected shoulder *if* the shoulder joint is not very carefully positioned. As illustrated in Figure 14, *the arm has been correctly placed well forward* and the shoulder is in an excellent position. If this is not done, the patient's body will roll on to the affected arm, trapping the shoulder in a wrong and very painful position that will build up much future trouble for the poor unfortunate patient and shortly turn arm rehabilitation into a disaster. Also, in this position the sound leg rolls over the affected leg as shown in the diagram. This serves a double purpose; it maintains an acceptable degree of mild internal rotation in the affected hip while, at the same time, it allows the affected hip to be held straight; whereas, in all other positions it is bent. The hip must be straight for part of each day, otherwise it will become stiff and cause problems later. As illustrated, it is possible for the patient to lie with it quite straight while the considerable degree of bend in the knee and the mild hip rotation will prevent any build-up of spasticity.

4. *Bridging*, as illustrated in Figure 15, ought to be included in any list of good bed positioning and also as one of the first exercises in self-care that the patient will be taught. As a starting position, it is taught for use in back lying where arms are correctly positioned and both legs are bent with knees together and feet planted firmly on the bed. To begin with, the patient will need careful teaching and help with this starting position and with the active exercise of 'bridging'. It is called bridging because the patient lifts his buttocks off the bed to make a bridge as illustrated. For obviouis reasons, it may be necessary to use bridging to assist early nursing. As a starting position, the patient is taught to lie on his back with arms correctly

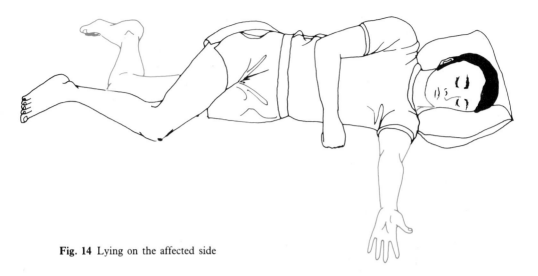

Fig. 14 Lying on the affected side

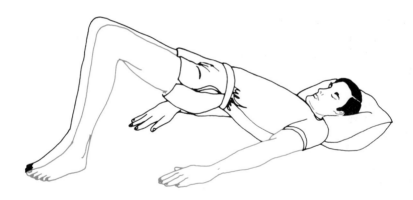

Fig. 15 Bridging

positioned and both legs bent up with knees together and feet planted firmly on the bed. At first the helper usually finds she has to help the patient to place and hold his affected foot and knee in the required position and he may also need assistance to lift his hips. Note, also, the illustrated arm position. The affected shoulder is well positioned and it is only the *lower arm* that is rolled inwards. In this position, when the patient lifts his hips, the resulting increase of pressure on his forearms and hands starts important weight-bearing and, at the same time, increases the roll outwards of the shoulders. If you find this point confusing, try the exercise on yourself.

A large, awkward or confused patient may need the assistance of two helpers, one on either side of the bed with a single handgrip under the small of his back to help him to lift. Or, if bed-pan nursing is needed, the first helper continues to hold the affected leg in position while the second helper uses her free hand to place the bed-pan in position. Bed-pan nursing is often not necessary where the patient is allowed by the doctor to sit out of bed from the beginning. Even so, bridging and all the bed exercises suggested in this book ought to be used in the early days while positioning for rest periods *must* be used meticulously. This is because it must at no time be forgotten that positioning must be used to help the patient to control his stronger reflexes so as to prevent developing spasticity while, at the same time, he is taught to follow many of the movement patterns we have learnt from watching the human infant's progress towards controlled movement.

So, why use bridging? Bridging *ought to be used* and firmly established as an early exercise. There are three clear reasons for making this statement.

1. The crook-lying position, lying on the back with knees bent up, is the position used to prevent build-up of the spasticity pattern which would force the affected leg out into full extension (or make it rigidly straight) if the patient spent time lying on his back with bad positioning. For this reason, the crook-lying position *must* be taught to the patient in the early days after the onset of his stroke. The knees are held firmly together, both pointing straight up to the ceiling to prevent the affected hip from rolling outward into the forbidden pattern. In the beginning, to help to establish the position, the patient may be taught to hold a book between his knees.

2. As soon as the patient has learnt to maintain the crook-lying position, he must learn to bridge without assistance by lifting his own hips as shown in Figure 15. Early weight-bearing is essential in stroke rehabilitation if the patient is to be given a reasonable hope of returning to normal living. This is because weight-bearing works on the postural reflexes and it has already been shown that rehabilitation depends on this. This is the first exercise in early weight-bearing. Bridging, by lifting the hips off the bed, brings the trunk muscles on the affected side into action and so begins the first active exercise in hip control. Remember that gross movements, or primary trunk movements, are the first controlled movements to be re-educated.

3. As soon as the patient can use the exercise freely, it enables him to take his weight off his buttocks at frequent intervals, maintaining comfort and reducing any risk of developing pressure sores.

Note. In my experience, any patient who fails to establish strong and controlled bridging in the treatment programme fails in later stages to establish full hip control and a normal walking pattern is never regained. Bridging also plays an important part in preparation for standing up and sitting down.

These three points about the usefulness of bridging set the pattern for the stroke rehabilitation programme. Successful rehabilitation is founded on a logical sequence of events. A list of the points made so far that ought to be remembered if the treatment programme is to be understood might help here.

1. Trunk movements return first and recovery spreads downwards, trunk to hip to knee to foot, and trunk to shoulder to elbow to wrist to hand. Any initial finger grip the paralysed arm may show will be a primitive movement that ought not to be encouraged. This means *do not*, at this stage, give the patient a ball to grip.

2. Positioning is used to prevent the build-up of unwanted reflex activity (or spasticity) and wherever possible the patient ought to be taught to maintain correct positioning for himself. In other words, it is a great help if it is possible to hand over the care of his own limbs to the patient himself. This is done by taking diligent care with early positioning, by explaining the reasoning behind the need for this diligent care, by supplying adequate supporting pillows and correct furniture and by offering every possible help to make it possible for the patient to maintain the required positions. For example, as suggested above, he may be taught to grip a book between his knees until he has learnt to hold the crook position, or he may be taught to clasp his hands with his palms touching and his arms outstretched to maintain the necessary arm position. This will be more fully described later.

3. As already stated, early weight-bearing is a must where controlled movement is to be re-educated. As rehabilitation progresses, greater weight-bearing demands will be made.

This leads to another question. *Is early weight-bearing for the shoulder necessary?*

It most certainly is. Turn back to Figure 2 and it will be seen that the infant weight-bears from elbow to shoulder at an early date in movement development. As the treatment programme unfolds it will be shown that weight-bearing through the arm plays a vital role in arm recovery. The arm must have very special attention if the paralysed patient is to be given any hope of regaining a useful hand. Bed exercises for the affected arm must begin as soon as possible after the onset of the stroke. This means that arm exercises do not immediately include weight- bearing but quickly lead up to propping on the elbow — or weight-bearing from elbow to shoulder. To begin with it helps if all joints of the hand and arm are given passive movements daily — that is, the helper moves the small joints, and then the limb as a whole, but this must include *keeping within the recovery pattern* and should not be attempted on the shoulder joint *if* this statement is not properly understood.

Figures 16, 17 and 18 show very clearly the necessary initial exercises that ought to be carefully used, at no time neglecting to keep the arm in the anti-spasticity (or recovery) pattern while the exercises are performed. *Note:* While all these exercises are performed the patient's pelvis, hip and knee on his affected side must be carefully positioned.

Figure 16 pinpoints the need to understand the correct pattern of movement for the shoulder joint — in other words, the starting position of the shoulder joint for this exercise is external (or outward) rotation and this position must be maintained while the arm is raised above the head. If in any doubt about this vital shoulder position, refer once more to Figures 8 and/or 12. In both cases external (or outward) rotation of the shoulder is quite clearly shown. Note that the thumb is pointing away from the body. If this correct positioning of the shoulder is fully maintained while the arm is raised above the head, at the end of the exercise the thumb should still point away from the body (as clearly illustrated in Fig. 16). The helper supports the elbow with one of her hands and by interlacing the fingers of her other hand with the patient's fingers she also helps to maintain the full recovery pattern. This particular pattern, external rotation of the shoulder with full elevation of the arm is a position which many people who care for stroke patients fail to establish. It is all too easy to start the movement correctly, palm facing upward and thumb pointing away from the body, but as the arm is raised above the head the shoulder is allowed to rotate into the forbidden spasticity pattern of internal rotation. The only way to make quite sure that the vital external rotation of the shoulder is maintained throughout the movement is to watch the thumb's position and keep it pointing steadily away from the body (as in the starting position) during the whole movement. Do not force the movement. Only raise the arm as high as it goes with comfort.

The shoulder of the stroke patient will give tremendous trouble and *very severe pain* if it is badly handled. As already stated, correct positioning from the very beginning is particularly vital for the rehabilitation of this particular joint. Wrong and careless positioning, as well as reinforcing any tendency to spasticity, will lead to trouble for two reasons:

1. The structure of the joint is such that, with handling in wrong positions, bony structure meets bony structure and the joint capsule and ligaments that surround the joint are involved in a very painful pinching or nipping.

2. Bad, or wrong, positioning leads to contraction of muscles round the joint and an immobile or stiff shoulder blade and the consequent pain caused by this stiffness. The pain of a stiff joint can be very severe.

Figure 17, arm raising, shows how the patient may do this most

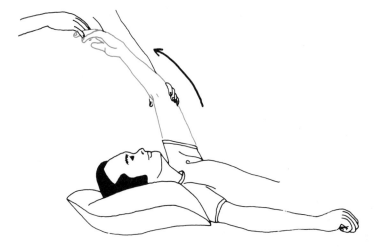

Fig. 16 Arm raising with external (outward) rotation

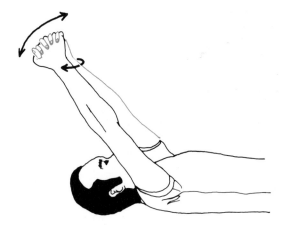

Fig. 17 Arm raising — self- care

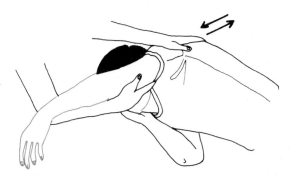

Fig. 18 Very necessary shoulder movements

important exercise of arm raising for himself. He must be taught to clasp his hands, *palms touching,* and to raise both arms as illustrated. An acceptable degree of external rotation of the shoulder is maintained by the clasped hands provided he keeps his palms touching. He may also be taught to turn his hands in the direction indicated by the circular arrow. **This exercise is very important.** A freely mobile shoulder must be maintained and, where self-care can be taught and used to assist rehabilitation, it will do the utmost good. It may help the reader if a list of reasons is given to show why this is an ideal self-care exercise.

1. It helps the patient to bring the affected hand into his mental picture of a whole body.

2. It helps him to be aware of its feel and of its position in space.

3. It uses the primitive reflex movement already shown in the baby — pushing his head backward as he lifts his arms helps him to straighten his affected arm.

4. It works the affected arm in the full recovery pattern and, as he can also do this exercise when he is sitting up, it may be repeated by him many times a day.

5. As a self-care exercise it gives the patient the satisfaction of doing something useful for himself. He will greatly assist the maintenance of shoulder mobility.

Figure 18, a very necessary shoulder movement, gives a very clear picture of how to help the patient to maintain a freely mobile shoulder. This is not a self-care exercise and the handgrips the helper should use are carefully illustrated. The arrows indicate the direction of movement and the movement keeps the shoulder blade freely mobile. It is important to remember that if the patient develops a painful shoulder during the early days after the onset of the stroke, those who are caring for him should look for two possible causes and correct any mistakes that are being made. These causes may be:

1. The patient has not been handled with due care and correct positioning has not been maintained.

2. The arm is not being placed, maintained and moved in the necessary anti-spasticity positions and internal rotation of the shoulder with trapping of the arm below the body has been allowed.

One night of lying in a bad position will trigger off the characteristic pattern of the agony shoulder that may be found in so many unfortunate stroke victims. Hence the urgent need to pay meticulous attention to the care of the shoulder.

Are there any other early bed exercises the patient ought to do?

Yes, early care of the shoulder has been shown but the hip must have as much help as possible if recovery is to go forward and normal movement is to be established. It has already been shown that careful positioning must begin immediately after the stroke and that the hip must therefore at all times be maintained in a bent position with special care taken to see that the leg is not allowed to roll outwards. Bridging has also begun and has been seen as a hip exercise. It should now be said that the crook-lying position which is taught for bridging should also be used as the starting position for hip rotation movements. In other words, the legs will be bent up in the crook-lying position with the knees held firmly together, the helper supporting and assisting the exercise where necessary, and both knees are moved together, rolling from side to side.

Figure 19 illustrates an exercise which ought not to be left out. The need to keep the hip bent to prevent build-up of spasticity means that it may later be difficult to straighten it properly in standing up. Bridging helps to prevent this from happening but the exercise, as illustrated in Figure 19, is also useful for the same reason. The leg is placed over the side of the bed and, in this position, the hip is straightened right out while passive knee exercises are easily given.

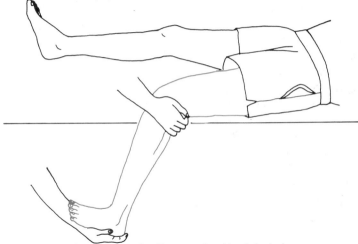

Fig. 19 Full hip extension with knee bending over the side of the bed

Figure 20, early weight-bearing on the affected foot, also illustrates another useful exercise which many patients achieve quite easily. Pushing down on the affected foot and raising the affected hip (however little) gives a strong and effective exercise. Remember that bed exercise sessions in these early days should not be too strenuous, should not be painful because bad positioning is the position of pain, and ought to stimulate the patient's interest with thoughts of recovery.

Positioning is the most important need and it must never be allowed to lapse or to be neglected.

Figure 21 shows the last of the important positions for use in bed. Before the patient is allowed to get out of bed it may be necessary for him to sit up in bed. Careful positioning is again of the utmost importance. He should sit as upright as possible with his head and trunk in a line and his weight going equally through both buttocks. As illustrated in Figure 21, the shoulder is well forward in external, or outward rotation and the arm is well positioned. Some therapists might prefer to see the affected arm raised higher on more pillows. Both are acceptable as long as the outward rotation of the shoulder is maintained. It is shown how a pillow is used to lift the affected hip slightly forward, keeping the leg from rolling outward into external rotation and the knee lies comfortably in slight flexion. A footboard or box *must not be used* to support the feet. This is because the forepart of the affected foot would press downward on the box and immediately start the unwanted reflex action of thrusting downward using the anti-gravity muscles strongly and triggering off unwanted spasticity. (For the same reason a leg calliper to support the knee and inevitably to put pressure on the ball of the foot should not be ordered for the patient in an attempt to stimulate early walking.) Note, also, that every time the patient turns towards the table or locker at the side of his bed he is rolling round, turning his shoulders against his pelvis which remains still. Once again he is using

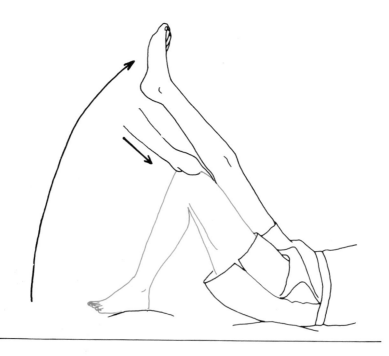

Fig. 20 Early weight bearing on the affected foot

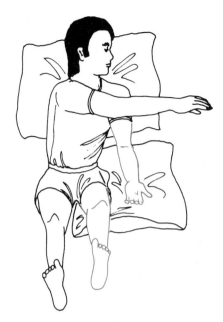

Fig. 21 Rolling the shoulders to reach across to bedside table

The human infant spends the first months of his life developing controlled movement

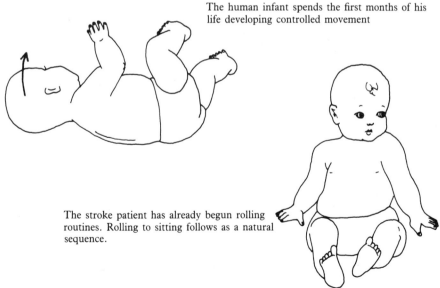

The stroke patient has already begun rolling routines. Rolling to sitting follows as a natural sequence.

Fig. 22 Rolling leads to controlled sitting

the baby's pattern of rolling (Fig. 22) and this kind of rotation also stops any leg spasticity because the hip rolls inward with the knee slightly bent. This position of sitting up in bed will probably not be used very much because usually as soon as the patient is ready to sit up the doctor wants him to sit out of bed. But there is a place for it in rehabilitation and when it is used it must be used correctly. As illustrated and for the reasons given, the patient, unknown to himself, is doing a most useful exercise in rehabilitation. Every time he reaches across to his bedside table he is using the sound side of his body to rehabilitate his weak side. Physiotherapists call this 'cross facilitation' and this is quite a good example of what is meant by 'living in the recovery pattern'. If every action all through the day can be related to movement within this recovery pattern, and if careful positioning is maintained when the patient is at rest, rehabilitation should go forward well.

An alteration and another therapeutic approach to sitting upright in bed may be made by giving the patient a bed-table which is positioned across the bed so that he can lean forward supporting himself on both forearms which are placed on the table parallel to each other. Using this position he should also be taught to clasp his hands together with his fingers interlaced. He will use this hand clasp position frequently during rehabilitation (he has already used it for double arm raising while lying on his back) so the sooner it is thoroughly mastered the better. He frequently needs help to interlace his fingers in the early days and, at the same time, he must be carefully taught to press his palms firmly together to help him to maintain the correct anti- spasticity pattern as well as to help him to be fully aware of both hands.

One more point ought to be mentioned before moving on to the next exercise progression. As explained, *a footboard must not be used*. This serves to illustrate a lesson that must be learnt early in the treatment programme if there is to be a successful outcome. Early weight-bearing is necessary but it must be *over a correctly positioned base*. In this instance, the forepart of the foot pressing down on a footboard is not giving a correctly positioned base. This point will be carefully demonstrated later in the text.

Both these positions for sitting upright in bed give very good examples of helping the patient to help himself. For this reason he should be told why it will help his recovery to reach across to the table which is placed on the affected side of his body. Every time he helps himself to a drink of water, or fruit juice, or a cup of coffee or tea, or a tissue or a book, he is furthering his own rehabilitation *but the affected arm must be carefully maintained in the recovery pattern*. Anti-spasticity or recovery patterns are also called inhibiting patterns because they affect the distribution of the patient's muscle tone, inhibiting the build–up of excessive anti–gravity muscle tone.

The helper must see to this by placing the arm correctly with adequate support. (*Note*. Most stroke patients need to be encouraged to drink enough. Fluids are very necessary.) It would be much less effort for the patient if the bedside table were to be placed on his sound side but it would in no way help his rehabilitation. Indeed, it would actively prevent recovery by teaching him to compensate with his sound side and lead to a so-called recovery where he lives his life out as a disabled person using only one half of his body with increasing residual disability of his affected side.

Using the second position where he sits upright with a bed-table positioned across the bed, while he leans forward on his forearms he is taking weight from elbow to shoulder and has begun the essential early weight-bearing. The arms must be parallel so that the affected shoulder is prevented from turning into internal rotation and he is bearing weight on a correctly positioned base. Again, he is continuing his own rehabilitation. Or, where, once again in the same starting position, he leans on his forearms and clasps his hands so as to raise both hands above his head with his arms outstretched (elbows straight) again he is furthering his own rehabilitation. He will probably readily understand why he must help himself to maintain a mobile shoulder.

As well as these early bed exercises passive movements should be given to the affected limbs at least twice daily. Passive movements are movements which are done by the physiotherapist or helper and the patient takes no active part. *But* correct movement patterns must be used, that is, the movements ought to keep within the anti-spasticity patterns. If the shoulder is kept in external or outward rotation, passive movement should not hurt. It must be remembered that in many cases the patient is having to relearn the movement — his brain has forgotten movement patterns and correct patterns ought to be re-established as soon as possible. Incorrect and trick movements are quickly learnt and, if this is allowed to happen, it will be found later that wrong movement patterns are impossible to discard. Treatment by exercise must include active as well as passive movement. Treatment progresses in three clear stages:

1. Passive movements in which the patient takes no active part.

2. Active assisted movements in which the patient actively assists his helper to produce the required movement.

3. Active movements in which the helper takes no part except, where necessary, to correct the patient's positioning or to support a limb in the correct position so that the required movement is possible.

Only active movement can give the patient the sensations that are necessary for re-education of voluntary movement and so the patient's active co-operation must be added to the helper's work with the affected limbs as soon as possible. At no time must the patient be allowed to make an excessive effort — this will only lead to build up of spasticity. As might be expected, the hip and shoulder joints will lead the way in this active co-operation. For example, if the patient is lying in bed and the helper is giving passive hip movements by bending and stretching the leg she will quickly move on to the stage where she asks her patient to 'help me to bend your hip'. Movement should be done slowly and the patient should be allowed plenty of thinking time. 'Now help me to bend your hip' is a command that may be very helpful. Passive movements to the hand should be given as often as possible and should include bending and stretching of the wrist and bending and stretching of all the finger joints, each joint to be moved separately and then the hand as a whole. These hand movements must only be done passively in these early days and any attempt on the patient's part to assist in bending will increasae any tendency to spasticity. Remember that the patient *must not* be asked to 'hold' a ball in his hand. Moving the joints passively to keep them from becoming stiff and immobile will later be a tremendous help when it comes to hand rehabilitation and re-education of active hand movements. These passive movements to the joints of the hand ought not to be left out of any treatment programme. Careful instructions should be given to all relatives who care for stroke patients at home. So far, the necessary bed positions have been shown and the caring relative, by following the text and diagrams, ought to be able to master these positions and to understand the harm that will be done if they are not used.

Where a domiciliary physiotherapist comes to the patient's home to teach the sequence of rehabilitation exercises and to lead the way in helping him to help himself towards independence, the caring family member is well advised to watch and learn all she can from the therapist so that she may be able to help by maintaining the same movements and patterns for living as used in rehabilitation. When the patient is in hospital it is to be hoped the hospital has a scheme going whereby the families of stroke patients are encouraged to become thoroughly involved in his care.

In a very small minority of cases the pattern of spasticity may not follow the pattern which is represented in this book. Here the physiotherapist must assess the pattern presented very carefully and advise any family member who works with her as to the slight alterations in positioning that may be necessary. Remember, this only applies to a very small minority. Otherwise, the spasticity patterns as presented in this book are the patterns that may normally be expected. We are dealing with anti-gravity muscles and of these, two main muscles must never be forgotten:

1. There is a very large and powerful muscle (strongly used when the gibbon pulled himself up into his tree) which pulls the shoulder downwards, backwards and inwards. (For those who want to know its name it is *Latissimus dorsi*.) To counteract this pull the patient's shoulder must be maintained by careful positioning in the opposite pattern — upwards, forwards and outwards.

2. The large bulk of the buttock is the biggest of the buttock muscles (*Gluteus maximus*) which extends the hip against gravity into the upright position and turns the leg outwards. Again it is to counteract this dominant anti-gravity pull that hip care is so important.

If those who care for the stroke patient realise the supreme importance of extra careful positioning for these two main joints, shoulder and hip, the patient will be faithfully started on the road to independence. It is proposed now to continue the text to cover the steps that are taken to help the stroke patient to regain independence. The exercises will be demonstrated by a physiotherapist (as will be shown in the diagrams) but only those exercises which may be faithfully copied by a friend or relative — or which may be done by the patient by himself with no help — will be included. Helpful explanatory notes will be given and it is hoped that the book may be used as a guide to help families to help their stroke patients to return to independence. With help the patient must learn how to maintain the essential inhibiting patterns and how to live within the recovery pattern. What is meant by living within the recovery pattern will become more apparent as the text advances.

Many patients are treated at home, or return home long before rehabilitation is completed, and treatment must continue along correct lines if the correct beginning is to go forward and offer a reasonable return to normal living. Where the disability is severe the patient will most probably be treated in hospital. It is to be hoped there will be a physiotherapist in attendance when he returns home and that she will teach and encourage the relatives as well as her patient.

It must be realised that no two stroke patients are exactly the same, or demonstrate exactly the same difficulties. There may be a tendency to severe spasticity with greatly increased tone in the anti-gravity muscles, or the limbs may be floppy and very heavy with greatly diminished muscle tone, or there may be a mixture of both, or even a tremor that occurs with some movements. There may be very severe loss of movement, or only slight loss, giving severe disability or only slight disability, nor should it be forgotten that things may be further complicated by sensory loss. This may include loss of awareness of the affected limbs and the patient may have lost his 'joint and muscle sense' and have no idea where his limbs are in space, or he may not even recognise that there is anything wrong with them. There may be speech or language problems which may also range frome mild to severe difficulty or may even go undetected and yet, at the same time, cause the patient much distress. Or, again, some of the most difficult problems of all may be present because of difficulty in the areas of the brain associated with conscious recognition and learning and memory. A patient may, for example, have very little loss of movement but be unable to use a spoon because he does not recognise it or have any idea what it is for. Or he may be quite unable to dress himself and if he is bullied he may try and put his trousers on his head. The various difficulties will be isolated by the specialists. How is it possible to give an outline of necessary rehabilitation practices if the difficulties encountered can be so many and varied? I believe the answer is quite simply that the modern approach to rehabilitation of the stroke patient, going right back to birth and following the patterns of movement and sensory development as seen in the human infant, must be the best possible answer as long as careful *inhibiting* positioning is used throughout. This will help the recovery of all stroke patients and the end result for each case will be the best that can be obtained for his degree of brain damage. After all, the infant does not speak before he stands up, he does not dress himself before he comes to terms with his environment and the specialist in neurology tells us that, whatever the brain damage, in time messages will get through. There are always other pathways. Why not set out to re-educate from the beginning? There is no good reason that can be given for rejecting this idea and there are many good reasons for adopting it. In my own case, the best reason I can give for adopting the method suggested is a high rate of success over many years of caring for stroke patients. I would add that it must be remembered where speech or language difficulties are involved *it is essential* to seek the help and advice of the speech therapist.

By using careful positioning, rehabilitation has made a good beginning. Let us take heart and continue the programme.

Accepting stroke illness and the disability it brings is not easy but, approached as suggested here, the patient will be given the best possible chance of making the most of his recovery and it is surprising how often the best is acceptably good. Also, approached in this way, disability is not increased by the onset of crippling spasticity and the patient and his family can expect to see some degree of favourable progress. Progress brings optimism and the cheerful spirit that is so necessary to recovery.

Where the patient is nursed at home from the beginning, the early days of home care may be exhausting for the caring family member and, where possible, the duties ought to be shared. Very soon the doctor will allow the patient to get up. Getting up does not mean he stops his bed positioning and exercises. They continue to be necessary and positioning should be meticulous until controlled movement is regained. Getting up itself will also be done as a therapeutic exercise where careful positioning continues and the patient is taught to work with the sound side of his body moving across (or rolling) to his affected side so as to initiate movement of the affected side. No activity is given without giving a thought to the effect it will have on the body as a whole — even watching television becomes an exercise in rehabilitation! The patient learns to live in the pattern of recovery. In this way, early independence is gained, self-respect is re-established and the patient becomes a whole person again. He begins by learning how to get himself out of bed.

Rolling leads to controlled sitting: Figure 22

First of all, then, rolling must be carefully taught until it becomes a controlled exercise. To a certain extent, rolling has already begun by turning the patient from side to side for nursing purposes and to obtain comfortable and correct sleeping positions. But, as far as recovery of active movement is concerned, turning from side to side has a vital part to play in the patient's recovery. This is simply because recovery of controlled movement takes place first in the movements of the trunk and, as in the case of the infant, the primitive movements involved in trunk rotation are the first to be involved in the plan to re-educate controlled movement from spinal reflex level upwards. If this is not understood it does not matter; just think of the infant and remember how he developed. Properly controlled, this turning or rolling movement helps the patient to be aware of both sides of his body and to use the affected side actively; it helps to initiate active movement in the shoulder and hip, recovery of the limbs starting in the shoulder and the hip. When rolling from side to side is taught, the important thing to remember is that the affected shoulder must be brought well forward and *must not be trapped under the body*. As soon as possible, turning from side to side ought to be encouraged as an active exercise. This is done by encouraging the patient to use the self-care arm position he has already learnt — hands clasped together, fingers interlaced, palms touching, elbows straight and reaching both arms above his head (Fig. 17) — and then to lead the movement by turning his eyes, his head and his hands in the direction of the turn.

Figure 23, rolling to the sound side, shows the initial help that may be needed to achieve the required result. Turning to the sound side (which means leading with the affected side) is much more difficult than turning to the affected side. Initially it may also help if the patient starts with his legs in the crook position he has already learnt. The helper should always stand on the side of the bed to which her patient is turning. This will increase his effort and remove any fear of falling.

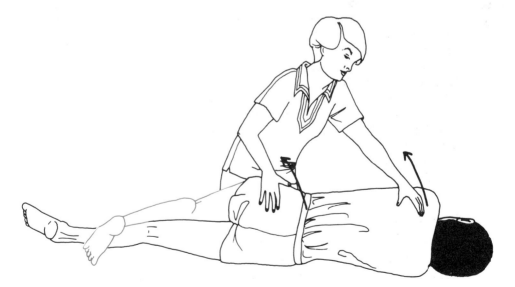

Fig. 23 Rolling to the sound side

Figure 24, rolling to the affected side, shows a progression to be made when rolling has been established. It demands a little more effort and prepares the way for the next exercise.

Figure 25, rolling to prop on the affected elbow, is an exercise which the stroke patient ought to practice and establish at an early date. The sooner he can master it the better because it is the next progression in learning to get himself out of bed and it is also a very important shoulder rehabilitation exercise. Again we mimic the infant's early movement pattern of rolling to elbow propping. As shown in Figure 25, the patient is encouraged to sit up with a sideways roll so that he finishes the movement by propping on his affected elbow. It is usually not difficult to establish this position, it just takes time and understanding encouragement. The helper holds the patient's affected elbow firmly in its correct resting position on the bed with her hand (as illustrated) while she uses her other hand to give a handshake (or cross) grasp to assist him, with a cross pull, to raise himself on to the affected elbow. If the starting position is correct, the elbow will be weight-bearing directly below the shoulder (as illustrated), *not behind the shoulder*. This is an important detail as it ensures correct shoulder positioning. The patient should then be encouraged to balance on the elbow before he is lowered gently back on to the bed. With each exercise session the exercise

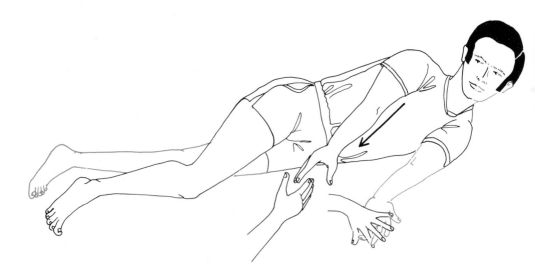

Fig. 24 Rolling to the affected side

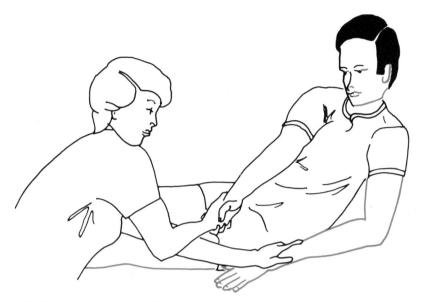

Fig. 25 Rolling to prop on the affected elbow

should be repeated several times so that the patient gets the feel of the movement. The object is to practise until he is able to elbow prop as described without the assistance of his helper. He then uses the movement every time he turns to reach out to the locker or table at the side of his bed. This is why the locker must be placed on his affected side. If it is placed on his sound side he simply uses the sound side of his body and ignores his weak side. This means he does not carry out the infant development pattern of rolling to propping and he does not recover his lost function. Once this rolling to elbow propping is established, the patient is weight-bearing from elbow to shoulder and not only has the all important early weight-bearing for the arm begun, but, with the assistance of careful furniture positioning, self-care and self-rehabilitation take another vital step forward. If this exercise causes shoulder pain it almost certainly means that due care of shoulder positioning has not been given from the beginning and/or the arm is not being correctly positioned *forward* with the hand far enough away from the side of the body to give the correct starting position. One night of bad or careless positioning can very easily be followed by a day of pain.

Carefully managed much of the patient's rehabilitation will be done by the simple tasks he performs as part of his sadly curtailed daily pattern of living *but* recovery will depend on the careful teaching and maintenance of the right starting positions and the right movement patterns. Again, this is what is meant by living in the recovery pattern.

The diagrams show very clearly how the patient may be taught to progress to sitting with his legs over the side of the bed. Figure 26, rolling to cross the sound leg over the affected leg, simply continues the forward rolling movement. The patient is taught to move from lying to propping on the affected elbow (Fig. 25) to rolling to cross the sound leg over the affected leg in one continuous movement. Without a pause after rolling to prop on the affected elbow, he is taught to throw his sound leg over his affected leg (continuing the rolling movement) while his helper assists his movement into the upright position by continuing her support and cross pull with their handshake grasp. At the same time she quickly changes her other hand to support his affected heel. His affected arm straightens as illustrated and the helper completes the movement by lowering his legs over the side of the bed.

Figure 27 shows quite clearly what may happen if the cross pull does not quite come off and the patient fails to come upright as his legs swing over the side of the bed. At this early stage in rehabilitation it is wise where possible to have a second helper standing by to give extra assistance if necessary. As illustrated in Figure 27, the correct movement will still take place if the main helper continues to give the correct sideways pull to assist her patient to gain the upright sitting position.

As soon as the patient is sitting in the upright position with his legs over the side of the bed the helper transfers her hands to give shoulder support.

There is a rehabilitation rule which every physiotherapist uses extensively when she is treating her stroke patients. This rule, called *body alignment*, states that when the head is in the upright position the body follows the head. This is the result of reflex action and is one of the reasons the infant manages to attain balance in the upright position. In stroke rehabilitation, where normal reactions are disturbed, the physiotherapist depends largely on the use of the patient's eyes and a correctly placed mirror to help her to help her patient to use body alignment to achieve an upright posture. For this reason, at this stage a mirror may be used to advantage as follows:

Where rolling to sitting causes any problems the second helper will be positioned on the other side of the bed (or even kneeling up on the bed) and may be needed initially to give support to the patient's shoulders and to assist the lift and turn into sitting. The second helper will then keep her position behind the patient with her hands held firmly on his shoulders so as to assist his sitting balance while the first helper places, or holds, a mirror in front of him so that he can see himself. The mirror ought to be at least large enough to give him a clear view of his head, neck, shoulders and upper trunk. His helper should give him a firm, clear command: 'Look at yourself in the mirror!' This is quite often followed by a quite spectacular involuntary response. He holds his head high, straightens his shoulders and stretches his trunk. The second helper may then assist his sitting balance by continuing to support his shoulders and pushing him gently and firmly in any direction while he continues to look in the mirror and is firmly told: 'Don't let me move you!' Frequently he shows a tendency to fall over to the affected side and gentle but firm pressure on his opposite side will help

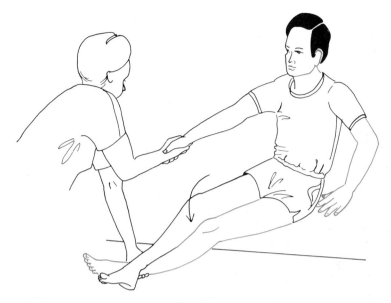

Fig. 26 Rolling to cross sound leg over affected leg

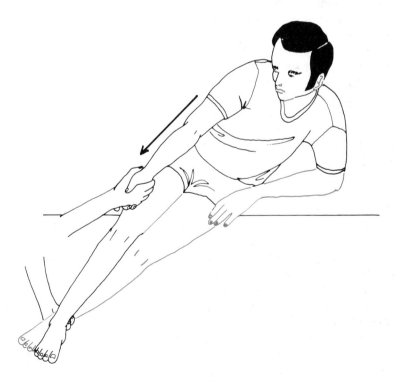

Fig. 27 Rolling to elbow propping to sitting, feet over the side of the bed

him to maintain sitting balance — or the upright position. A second helper should not be necessary for long.

Figure 28 demonstrates very clearly how the helper works when she is alone and not using the mirror. The method of sitting up as described here is a progression from simple rolling. This might be a suitable place to point out once again that the patient's rehabilitation programme depends on constant repetition of exercises which lead forward by easy progressions through a carefully planned pattern — the pattern following the infant's motor development where rolling leads to sitting. The moment sitting is achieved, training of sitting balance must begin. Frequently it will not be established at once. In the ideal situation, the correct height of bed for training sitting balance is the height which allows the patients to sit with his knees at right angles and his feet firmly on the floor. If this is not possible, a wooden box or footstool may be used to give the same effect.

When sitting balance is thought to be established the helper may gently withdraw her hands while she continues to support his knees with her knees as illustrated. If her patient then shows that balance has not been successfully established, she promptly reinforces her supporting pressure with her hands, then withdraws it very slowly from his weak side while she increases it very slowly on his strong side. The supporting pressure must be used carefully and gently to help the strong side of the patient's body to follow his head into the upright position. At no time ought the exercise to turn into a battle of strength and an increase in pressure ought to be given slowly to allow time for the desired reaction to take place. Following this method, sitting balance is usually fairly quickly established provided early treatment is given. But, in some cases it is necessary to move on to the next stage — getting from the bed to a chair — before the patient is thoroughly stabilised in sitting.

Figure 29, transfer from bed to chair, shows a very good method for helping the patient to perform this movement when upright sitting balance has not been fully established. In this case it is necessary to give the patient the maximum support while he transfers to the chair, at the same time allowing him to use the fully functioning half of his body. From this illustration it will be seen how necessary it is to have the chair correctly positioned before making the move. If in doubt, consult Figure 9b. The chair must be in the correct position so that all that is required of the patient is one easy movement — standing up and sitting down with a quick quarter turn. As shown in Figure 29, the helper is using her knees to support her patient's knees. She is supporting his affected arm, she is encouraging him to lean forward into standing by supporting his back and letting him make full use of the sound half of his body by placing his sound arm round her shoulders and standing up to full weight-bearing on his sound leg with supported weight-bearing on his affected leg. Properly carried out, this is a safe and easy way for a stroke patient to begin getting up. Leaning forward is a necessary part of standing up and, handled in this

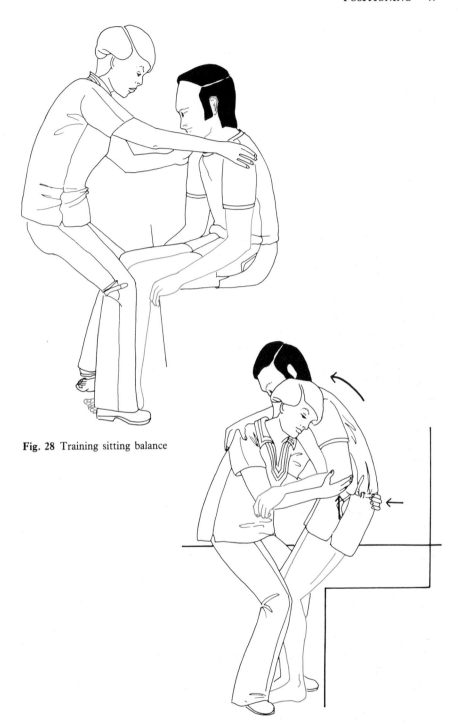

Fig. 28 Training sitting balance

Fig. 29 Transfer from bed to chair

way, it is easy to teach him to lean forwards, to stand up, to give a quarter turn and to sit down in the chair. The importance of placing the chair in the correct position will now be understood.

Figure 30 shows the patient sitting using his cantilever table. The red stripe of sticky tape down the middle of the table is put there to remind him that his affected hand must not be allowed to cross it and rest on the other side of the table. The moment his hand is allowed to cross this line his shoulder turns into the forbidden pattern of internal rotation. (Note that this is why a sling must not be used to support the affected arm.) There are those who say you cannot expect a patient to sit like this all day. The answer to this criticism must be that you can and must expect him to sit like this (unless otherwise correctly seated as will be shown later, or when he is standing) for every moment of his day *if* he is to maintain his painfree shoulder and if he is to rehabilitate his arm. By leaning on the affected forearm in this position he is weight-bearing over a correctly positioned base and he is rehabilitating his own arm. It is a question of early and careful training so that the correct position is readily accepted by the patient. Wherever possible, it is best to explain the reasoning behind this essential positioning and the patient's full co-operation is consequently obtained. A second table must be carefully positioned as shown in Figure 9b and c so that he must turn and reach across his body with his sound side every time he requires an article from the second table. Books, drinking water, fruit, the newspaper, pen and writing paper or whatever may be needed will then be placed to hand on this second table. Not cigarettes if it is possible to break a former smoking habit. Again the patient ought to be told that smoking will not lead to future good health.

Variations of this sitting position are shown in the photographs at the end of the book and in each picture it will be noted that the arm is carefully positioned with the forearm correctly supported.

Figure 31 has been included to show the use of a more difficult table; this is the type of table that is so frequently found in the hospital situation. The legs and cross-bar get in the way of the patient's correct leg positioning and unless it has a locking device it slides all over the place. It serves to demonstrate how infinitely superior the cantilever table is for use with the stroke patient. As illustrated in this diagram, the patient has obtained a degree of stability and control of his shoulder and elbow and is practising a fairly advanced arm exercise which is usually placed much later in the programme. Again, it has been placed here to show that the top of the table is too small. It would not give adequate forearm and hand support for use all through the day. It is best to set out on rehabilitation using the best possible table (the cantilever). At this stage it will help if the patient is taught to clasp his hands and use his sound hand to rotate his affected hand so that the palm of his affected hand turns upwards to face the ceiling. This is another exercise in self-care. The affected forearm must stay on the left side of the red tape (if the stroke disability is on that side, as illustrated. The right arm would be kept on the right of the tape for right-sided disability.).

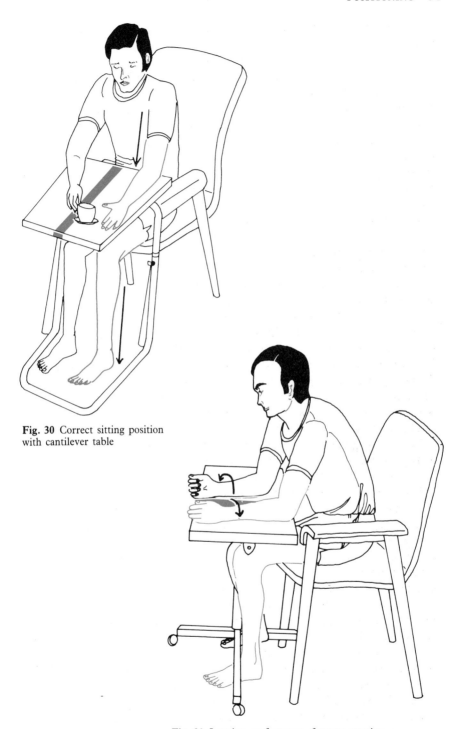

Fig. 30 Correct sitting position
with cantilever table

Fig. 31 Leaning on forearms, forearm rotation

Figure 32 once more demonstrates a rather unsatisfactory table in use. Here the raised edging on the table gets in the way of some of the rehabilitation practices and, once more, the top of the table is inadequate. Here the patient continues with the handclasp position and raises both hands above his head, as he did in bed (Fig. 17). Again he must be taught to keep his palms touching and the circular arrow indicates the direction in which he is taught to turn his hands. As illustrated, all is well with the arm

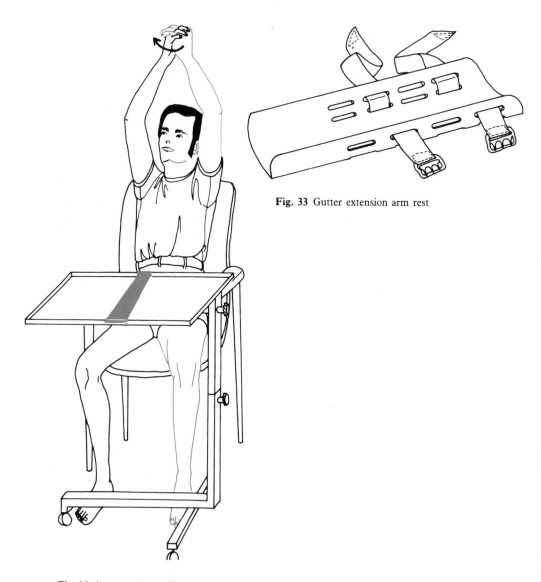

Fig. 33 Gutter extension arm rest

Fig. 32 Arm exercise, self- care

position but the patient has forgotten to control his leg position. He needs help to correct it. *His knees ought to be closer together* so that there is no danger of the affected hip rolling outwards. While sitting at his table he may be taught, as an exercise, to hold a book between his knees which must be bent to 90° with his *heels* firmly on the floor. While seated at his table he may be asked to slide his clasped hands forwards as far as possible and then lift them upwards to shoulder level and rotate his arms fully to right and left. This is done by turning his eyes, his head and his hands (in that order), moving from side to side in a wide sweep, maintaining the clasped hands at shoulder level.

Figure 33 shows a useful gutter extension arm rest. It may be strapped to the arm of the chair for forearm support when the table is not in use. It allows the patient to lean comfortably on the affected forearm so that he is weight-bearing from elbow to shoulder. When the gutter is in use for television viewing, make sure the television set is correctly positioned (Fig. 9c).

Sitting leads to controlled standing

Figure 34 has been included as a reminder that the simple development pattern of the infant is being closely followed. Do not expect the stroke patient to be able to control his sitting balance at once (any more than the infant could) and do not expect him to rise to balanced standing overnight!

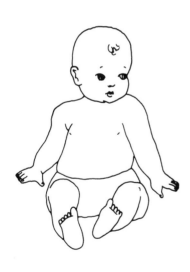
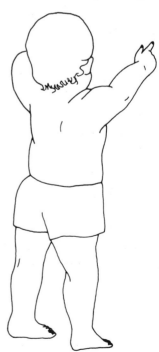

Fig. 34 Sitting to standing

Figure 35, training sitting balance, may take some time. On the whole it is not wise to attempt to achieve standing balance before sitting balance has been thoroughly mastered. Training in sitting balance (as already described) will be continued when the patient is sitting on the edge of the bed and also while he sits in the chair. Here a large mirror will help him to maintain an upright position if it is placed so that he can see his head and shoulders. When he is in the chair with his arm supported in the gutter extension and the mirror in place, he is ready for a training session. His helper will teach him to lean a little forward away from the back of the chair. Then she will ask him to look in the mirror and hold this good position while she gently pushes him in all directions. 'Don't let me push you', or 'Don't let me move you' may be the commands she uses while she slowly and carefully changes the position of her hands and the direction of her push. Her command would be, 'Don't let me turn you' when she uses both hands and gently tries to rotate his body. At all times during these important exercises the affected arm and leg *must* be very carefully positioned in the inhibiting pattern. If at any time the patient is seen to sag to one side into a poor sitting position, the helper should place one of her hands on the opposite side of his body and command him to 'Come on, push against me!' Again her pressure should be gentle but firm so that he comes upright into the correct position. He must be encouraged to make full use of the mirror.

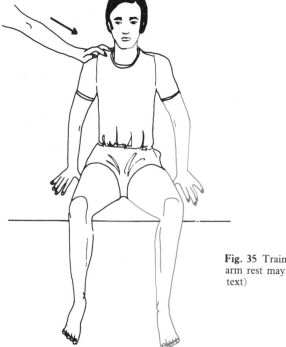

Fig. 35 Training sitting. Gutter extension arm rest may be used to advantage (see text)

Figure 36, standing transferring from bed to chair, is a progression on Figure 29. By now the patient has achieved a fair degree of sitting balance and is quite ready to use the sound side of his body to allow him to get in and out of bed safely with minimal help. As illustrated here, this is a fairly simple progression, and as soon as possible even this minimal help should be withdrawn so that he will have the satisfaction of managing for himself. He must be given the independence that is so necessary to boost morale. If his chair is correctly positioned at the side of his bed and he has been carefully trained in the correct and safe routines, he should not get into difficulty. At night the chair ought to be removed and an armchair commode put in its place. This will greatly assist return of bladder control where necessary and will give a tremendous boost towards return of any loss of self-respect.

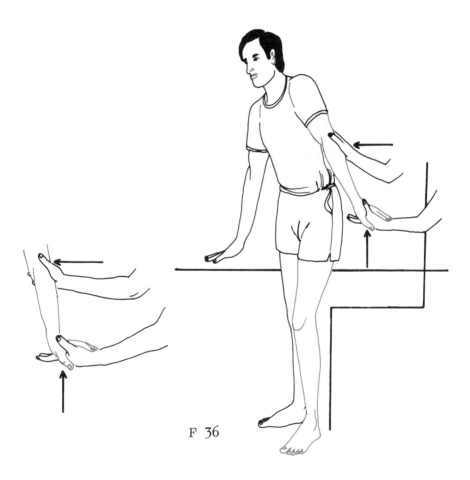

F 36

Fig. 36 Standing, transferring from bed to chair

Figure 37 shows how the helper may hold her patient's hand so that she can easily keep his arm in the recovery pattern — shoulder rolled outwards with his thumb pointing away from his body, palm facing forwards, and elbow straight.

Figure 38, preparation for standing from the chair, shows the patient with both of his hands resting on the arms of the chair. This has been included to emphasise that the patient must be taught to lean forwards and push on his hands to stand up. He must *push* to standing, not pull to standing. If he reaches forward to grasp an object and tries to pull to standing, he will only succeed in lying backwards and sliding out of his chair. A little pressure given by his helper on the front of his chest will help him to lean forwards and this may be followed by pressure on the back of his head in a forward and upward direction. If he is not ready to push to standing on both hands, the helper will take the affected hand as illustrated in Figure 36 and ask him to lean forwards and push on both hands. In this way she gives the necessary support to the affected arm.

Figure 39 shows how he ought to approach his chair (or commode) when he stands up to transfer from one to the other. Once more, this makes it quite obvious why the furniture must be correctly positioned. In the middle of the manoeuvre, before he moves his sound arm across to the second arm of the chair (or commode), he is taught to *take time* to make sure he is balanced and then to turn his feet a little in the direction of the turn before he transfers his hand in the direction indicated by the arrow. With his hand firmly in position on the second arm of the chair (or commode), he is ready to finish the turn by rotating his body and sitting down in safety. Very soon, as before, he will be able to carry out this transfer on his own.

Figure 40, standing up and sitting down, is included as a guide for those who find difficulty in training their stroke patient to achieve this stage in rehabilitation. The physiotherapist's approach as shown here demonstrates the need to teach the patient to *lean forwards*.

Figure 41, achieving equilibrium (or balance) with the aid of a rocking chair, shows one of the most useful aids in stroke rehabilitation. As shown,

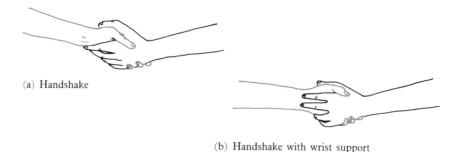

(a) Handshake

(b) Handshake with wrist support

Fig. 37 Two more useful handgrips to reinforce the recovery pattern

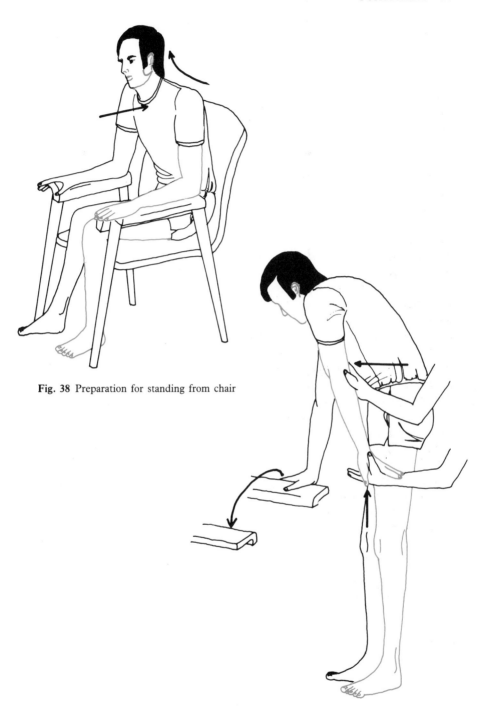

Fig. 38 Preparation for standing from chair

Fig. 39 Correct approach to chair before sitting down, or transferring from chair to commode

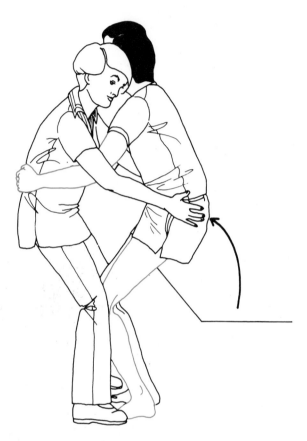

1st. Command: "Lean well forward . . . . . . and stand up!" The physiotherapist's body prevents the patient's affected arm from falling into the pattern of spasm, her arm grips and controls his elbow, her hand controls his hip, her knees control his knees. Alternatively both of his arms may be placed over her shoulders while her hands are placed over his shoulder blades.

2nd Command: "Lean well forward . . . . . and sit down!" The helper's weight counter-balances the patient's weight and the seesaw motion makes this an easy movement to accomplish.

Fig. 40 Standing up and sitting down

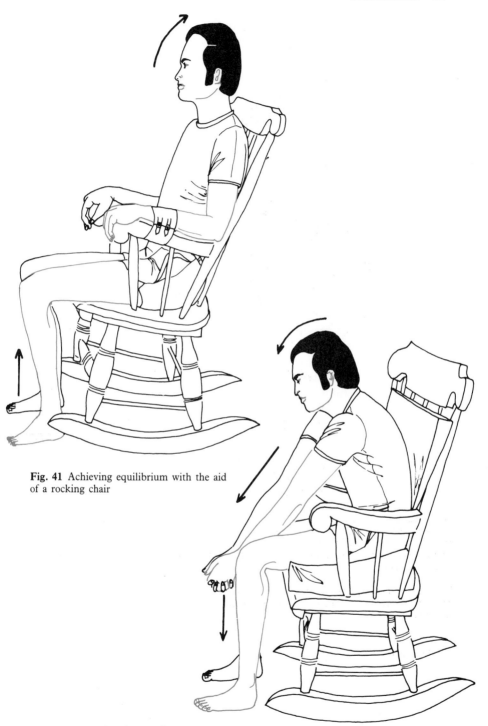

Fig. 41 Achieving equilibrium with the aid of a rocking chair

Fig. 42 Preparation for standing up

the patient is placed in a very good sitting position and he is weight-bearing through his heels to maintain the rocking movement. The affected leg must not be allowed to slide forward so that he weight-bears through the front part of his foot. This would use the unwanted pattern of the strong reflexes and would spoil the foundation he is carefully building so that he may shortly establish a good walking pattern.

Figure 42 shows how he uses the rocking chair to help towards leaning forwards for standing up. Again he is beautifully positioned and has incorporated a useful arm exercise into the correct rocking pattern. If the patient has short legs, for all rocking chair exercise it is usually necessary to give him a raised step to rest his feet on so that he is able to push down correctly on his heels and not on the front part of his feet. A small wooden box, a block of foam-rubber or a polystyrene step may be used, but whatever is used to make the step it must not get in the way of the chair's rockers.

Weight-bearing over a correctly positioned base

The need for early weight-bearing has already been stressed. The need to weight-bear over a correctly positioned base ought to be fully understood. Where possible, the reasoning behind this need for meticulous positioning ought to be explained to the patient himself. With understanding it very quickly becomes almost automatic to maintain the patient's limbs in the correct position and, in many cases, the patient himself will see that positioning is carefully maintained. The need to live in the recovery pattern becomes a habit rather than a tedious chore.

By now it must be clear that the necessary meticulous positioning includes the whole of the patient's body which must also include the position of a hand or a foot. The position of the weight-bearing base must be seen to have a direct bearing on the position of the body it supports. Also, when sitting, the patient must not be allowed to sit with his weight going through only one side of his body. He must have his weight evenly distributed through both his buttocks. This is one of the reasons why the importance of training sitting balance has been stressed. *The patient must be balanced over both buttocks;* he must sit on a correctly-positioned base. A correctly-positioned base must include the position of the affected arm and leg. Again, in sitting, the patient must support his weight through both forearms which are correctly positioned on the cantilever table in front of him, or through one arm correctly positioned; if it is only through one arm it ought to be the affected arm (Fig. 30). If the hand and forearm are correctly positioned the shoulder above will be correctly positioned. In the words of the physiotherapist, the shoulder will not be allowed to turn into the pattern of the dominant reflexes. In the same way, if the foot and thigh are correctly positioned, the hip will not be allowed to roll outwards into the dominant, or wrong, pattern. Correct positioning of the limbs has already been carefully explained. Also it has been suggested that it is equally necessary to weight-bear on the arm as well as the leg. As rehabilitation progresses, this weight-bearing includes more and more standing on the foot and it *must* include standing on the hand. Many people forget that to progress to standing on limbs that are not first carefully positioned frequently leads to the vital shoulder and hip joints turning into the wrong positions and *good* rehabilitation progress is halted. Again, in the words of the physiotherapist, the arm is mobilised into outward rotation and the leg is mobilised into inward rotation. Put simply, the position of the base will determine the position of the joints above and the position of these vital joints must be correct if maximal functional recovery is to take place. It might be helpful to suggest to the helper that she experiments with weight-bearing through her own limbs so that she may understand fully what happens when the weight- bearing base is altered.

Figure 43 illustrates the correct positions for weight-bearing on the hand and on the foot. The cross-hatching indicates the surfaces that take the weight, the arrows indicate the acceptable and the unacceptable rotation that may take place. The finger-tips take minimal weight; as with the foot, the heel of the hand must take the main weight. As shown in the illustration we are looking at the weight-bearing base from below upward. The heel of the hand and the heel of the foot are the two areas which play the greatest part in recovery of normal movement in stroke rehabilitation. Once again, in the words of the physiotherapist, weight-bearing through these areas is essential if primitive reflexes are to become fully integrated into controlled movement. Is it any wonder that positioning of these two vital areas is of prime importance?

Note. A block of firm foam rubber makes the best footstool to aid positioning of the affected foot. Both feet will be placed on the 'footstool' and it should be of the correct height to maintain the knee at 90° when the patient is sitting so that his weight rests through his heels (correctly positioned) and a deep **heel** imprint should show in the foam at the end of an exercise session. Again note that the 'footstool' must not get in the way of the chair's rockers where the rocking chair is used.

As rehabilitation progresses this weight-bearing through these two vital areas, *the heel of the hand and the heel of the foot,* will play an ever increasing part in the exercise programme. But it must not be forgotten that the position of these areas must be considered from the first days of getting out of bed — even while the patient learns to sit with his weight distributed through both buttocks (e.g. note positioning of the affected limbs in Fig. 30). In other words, it is equally important to sit and to stand with correct positioning of hands and feet because, at all times, the *correct positioning of the shoulder and the hip* must be maintained. The early handling and positioning of the patient can so easily make or mar the rehabilitation prospects. *Handing over the care of his own limbs to the patient himself* as quickly as possible ought to be the aim from the beginning. **He must live in the pattern of recovery.** If this is made possible for him by careful

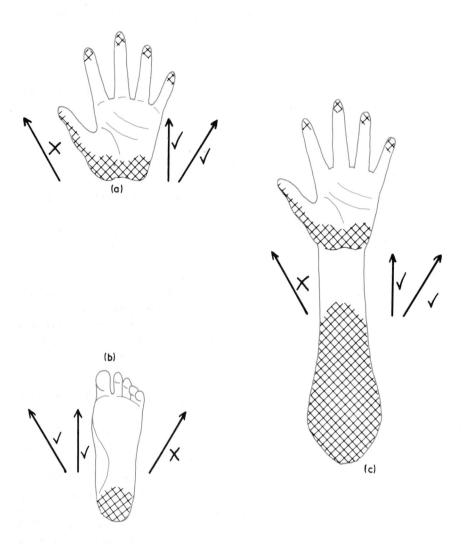

Fig. 43 Weight-bearing over a correctly positioned base on (a) the heel of the hand (b) the heel of the foot (c) the forearm and hand

teaching, by using correct methods of handling at all times, by using suitable and correctly placed furniture and by initial painstaking instruction in what must seem at times to be an almost obsessional attention to minute detail, as I have said, living in the recovery pattern becomes a habit rather than a tedious chore.

Summing-up

If the stroke patient is to live in the recovery pattern the following points must be understood, remembered and used:

1. Correct positioning of the patient at all times.
2. Correct positioning of the patient's furniture so that he is encouraged to assist rehabilitation by working across midline from the sound side of his body to the affected side.
3. All movement carefully follows the patterns of movement seen in the development of motor control in the human infant.
4. All movement must also take place within the recovery pattern, i.e. into the anti-spasticity pattern and away from the spasticity pattern.
5. The arm is mobilised into external rotation.
6. The leg is mobilised into internal rotation.
7. Weight-bearing will be used as much as possible but, at all times, this must include weight-bearing over a correctly positioned base.
8. Ways and means must be found to ensure that weight-bearing through a correctly positioned arm will be practised from the beginning and will not be allowed to lag behind weight-bearing through the leg.

As presented here, early mobilisation and the stages taken towards an early and very necessary move towards independence have taken all these points into consideration.

To those who say (and they are many) that you frequently get a fair degree of recovery in the affected leg of the stroke patient but recovery in the arm is minimal, I believe there is an answer.

I would say that it is a comparatively easy task to maintain the affected leg in the recovery pattern while sitting and to weight-bear over a correctly positioned foot. It is a relatively difficult task to sit with an arm that is constantly maintained in the correct position and it requires a great deal of ingenuity to do an adequate amount of weight-bearing through a correctly positioned forearm and hand and to *stand on a correctly positioned hand* in order to promote recovery. It is not surprising that in many cases it may be essential to seek the help of the physiotherapist and the occupational therapist in the planning of the early programme.

The patient may be faced by problems of speech or language. His customary method of communication with his fellow man may have been removed at a 'stroke'. He may be quite unable to make his needs understood and any problems in this field ought to be tackled at once. It is essential to establish some form of communication at once. *But this is a problem for the specialist* and the help of the qualified speech therapist ought to be sought at once.

Before continuing with the motor development patterns the patient may use to further his rehabilitation I therefore propose to seek the help of the specialist in problems of communication. She will attempt to shed light on this very difficult area and it will be seen that it is essential to have her assessment and advice before the unqualified helper or any other member of the rehabilitation team moves in to 'assist'. The *right* help is of paramount importance; the *wrong* help can all too easily be offered and can lead to disaster.

4   *Sandra Jackson Anderson*

Speech therapy

Probably one of the most appalling aspects of a stroke is that, for a few unfortunate patients, it can disrupt normal means of communication. Depending on the degree of severity, the patient may lose the power to understand speech, to read, to write and to communicate through words. One day to be healthy and the next to be paralysed is in itself an appalling experience. But, to find also that you have no means of communicating must be terrifying. The stroke patient, whose speech has not been affected, is able to ask all the questions for which he must have answers. Why did it happen? Will it happen again? What can you do for me? What does the future hold? In so doing, he is able to talk about his problems and alleviate his fears. The stroke patient who cannot speak often does not have these questions answered; he has no-one with whom to share his worries.

Immediately after the stroke he will feel very isolated, possibly depressed and even aggressive. Therefore, it is of the utmost importance that early on he is told what has happened and what we can hope for in the future. We must all be sensitive to his needs and anticipate the questions for which he must have answers. Although he cannot speak, or in some cases even understand, he is still the person he was before and should be treated as such. All those who have any dealings with him must explain what is being done for him and why. Even when we, the helpers, know that his ability to understand has been affected, we must still explain things to him slowly and clearly.

In the early days, the speech therapist may want to give intensive therapy herself, for at this stage it is often a job for the specialist. Only after the initial stages may she involve others in the direct treatment programme. However, that by no means implies that everyone else is redundant. Exercises alone do not bring back speech — *rehabilitating the desire to communicate* is the most important thing, and that is something which everyone must be involved in.

Never presume that because a patient is dumb he is also deaf for language. *Never hold conversations around him* — he must always be included no matter how severe his language problem. He has enough feelings of isolation within his own head without adding to them, and he needs all the support, communication and language stimulation that we can give.

Because he may feel isolated, it is therefore essential that he is not isolated from language. He needs normal conversation, albeit one-sided. However, this conversation may need to be modified according to the type of communication problem which the patient has. Therefore, an attempt will be made here to describe the different communication problems that may follow a stroke and the best way to approach them.

What are the communication problems?

The names given to disorders of communication following a stroke can be listed under three main headings:

1. *Dysphasia*

There are two basic types of dysphasia; receptive and expressive. With this problem, the patient's language function has been reduced due to damage of the speech centres in the brain. He may be unable to understand speech and therefore also cannot speak logically. Or, he may be unable to find the correct sound or words for speech even if his understanding has not been affected.

2. *Dyspraxia*

This is generally found in conjunction with dysphasia. The patient may be able to select the correct word from his brain, but the lips and tongue will not co-ordinate properly to form the letters. These two problems, *dysphasia* and *dyspraxia*, are in the majority of cases associated with a right-sided paralysis. This is because it is the left side of the brain which controls language, and it is that side of the brain which has been damaged.

3. *Dysarthria*

This is normally found in patients with a left-sided paralysis, and hence there is usually no language difficulty. The problem is purely at mouth level. The muscles are weak and because of this speech is slurred and unintelligible. But it should be noted that all patients with left-sided weakness do not necessarily suffer from dysarthria.

For the sake of clarity, these three disorders will be described separately. But it must be remembered that occasionally there can be a combination of speech disorders within the one patient. That, however, can be fairly complex and is best described to all who care for the patient by the speech therapist who assesses him.

Dysphasia

The two basic types are:

a. *Receptive dysphasia*

This is the most severe communication disorder. The patient's language as a whole — understanding, speaking, reading and writing has been drastically reduced. For better understanding, the reasons for this reduction in language can once more be subdivided under two headings:

(i) *Language input.* The patient may understand very little of what is said to him. A good example of this problem will be demonstrated if you can imagine that you know a foreign language, e.g. French, in that you have attained a basic vocabulary and no more than a fairly intermediate and limited level and someone starts speaking fluent French to you. You would know that he was speaking French, you would be able to pick up the occasional word and perhaps get the gist of the conversation, but you would be unable to comprehend fully what was being said. This is perhaps the best way to imagine a receptive dysphasia, but this may only apply after the patient has recovered a bit. In the dark days, immediately after his stroke, he may not realise that he has a language deficit and therefore may not be listening. Quite often the patient *thinks* that he is understanding and that he is speaking perfectly logically. He may do what he thinks you have just asked him to do and then be surprised to find you shaking your head in disagreement. Likewise, he may become frustrated if you do not obey his commands or answer the questions which he believes he is asking. It is not difficult to imagine how totally bewildering these early days must be.

(ii) *Language output.* This can take several forms, the patient can be speechless and on the whole totally oblivious to language, or he can have a recurrent utterance i.e., one word which he repeats over and over again e.g. 'do — do — do'. Sometimes it may sound like speech because the patient may use the inflexion and intonation of speech but, if you listen closely, it may be nonsense, letters and sounds all mixed up e.g. 'buddle toe swarmer me'. Lastly the patient may be speaking in English words, but the content is often meaningless and there may be no grammatical form e.g., 'may with house been was the are'. This is called jargon.

The most important thing to do initially with a receptive dysphasia, is to *ask the speech therapist to assess.* This will show just how much the patient is understanding, because quite often the level of understanding can be very deceiving. As has been previously stated, the patient is still the same person as he was before. He is not demented or confused, he knows where he is and what is being done for him, and, in the early days in hospital, he may need to use very little language comprehension because there is so much visual stimulation with visual cues.

For example, a normal morning routine may start with the nurse bringing the patient a basin of water and saying: 'Get your face-cloth and soap!' He does this, not necessarily because he understands what the nurse has said, but because it was the logical thing to do. She may then produce a shaving mirror and say: 'Get your razor!' (*Note*. An electric razor if the patient is using the non-preferred or unaccustomed hand.) Again he may do this because it is the next logical action in a chain of events. He may then be given his clothes, and here again, language comprehension may not be essential because he knows which garments to put on, albeit he may need help. So, on he may go to physiotherapy which is essentially physical, involving a great deal of gesture and visual cues. Here also, need for language comprehension may be minimal. (Frequently, in the early days of his second year, the human infant will carry out meaningful actions as a result of visual stimulation with visual cues while his understanding of language is still limited.)

Next, the patient may go on to speech therapy (in this case it is to be hoped that he does) and the speech therapist may discover that he can comprehend very little, and even finds difficulty in comprehending and obeying one simple command e.g. 'Give me the pen', because she has taken away all visual cues and is making him rely solely on language. When she reports this information to the team who care for him, they may be astonished. The nurse may say that, although he cannot speak, he understood her perfectly that morning and did everything she asked. However, if the nurse had gone through the procedure in reverse, she might have got a very different reaction. For example, if she had gone to the patient and simply said: 'I am going to bring you a basin of water and a shaving mirror, could you get your soap, towel and razor ready?', she might have returned to find that he had done nothing because he had not understood; or that he had done something bizarre such as producing his dirty washing, because he had put a different interpretation on what she had said, perhaps from getting the gist of washing but not the full meaning.

Thus it can be seen how important gesture and non-verbal cues (the basin and so on) are to communication. It is also very important to realise the value of gesture in the early days. The use of gesture reduces frustration and is a necessary means of communication. However, as the patient becomes stronger, he must be made to listen to language and to interpret verbal as well as non-verbal messages.

With a receptive dysphasia, the speech therapist is primarily interested in finding out exactly how much language the patient is understanding, and she has various assessments which she uses to ascertain this. She is looking for the answers to the following questions. Is her patient able to comprehend one simple sentence, or can he manage to understand two or more concepts at once? For how long can he concentrate? How accurate is his recent memory?

When the speech therapist has discovered the level at which the language breakdown is occurring, she can then advise the relatives on the best way in which to communicate with the patient. Going back to the earlier example of someone speaking French, imagine how much easier it would be, if instead of speaking the language fluently, it was spoken *slowly and clearly and simply*. This would make it much easier to follow. So it is *for the receptive dysphasic*. In this case, to some extent, the patient's own language is now foreign to him.

Concentration and memory may also be reduced and dysphasic patients may be unable to cope with more than one concept at a time. For example, suppose the patient is given four questions in one quick sentence: 'It's a lovely day, isn't it? Would you like a cup of tea? Will I move you over to the window to have it? Would you like to go to the toilet first?' Here his brain has to process these four questions that are tossed at him in rapid succession before he produces an answer. In general, this would be too much for the patient with receptive problems to cope with. He cannot cope for the following reasons:

a. *Language comprehension*: too much language all at once
b. *Concentration*: too many words and questions to be interpreted, he may lose interest
c. *Memory* he may forget one of the questions in his effort to interpret one of the others.

The above has been perhaps a slightly exaggerated example, but hopefully it illustrates how not to speak to such a patient. Therefore, how should you speak to him? Firstly, make sure you have his full attention; don't be afraid to touch his ear and say: 'Listen!' Then, very simply, one theme at a time, speak slowly and clearly. 'Would you like a cup of tea?' Give him plenty of time to interpret the question and indicate his answer. Then go on: 'Would you like to go to the toilet?' Again give him plenty of time. Lastly, without rushing: 'Would you like to sit by the window?'

These essential rules apply to all receptive dysphasic patients:

1. Get the patient's attention
2. Speak slowly and clearly
3. Only offer one idea or question per sentence.

This sounds fairly simple, but it is probably one of the most difficult things to put into practice. Remember that the patient is still the same person as he was before and most adults would be highly insulted to have you 'spell it out in words of one syllable'. So, while the theory behind this is very easy to understand, putting it into practice can be very difficult. Obviously, if you sound condescending or childish when you speak to him, your patient may be even more frustrated, feeling that you are treating him as if he is daft when he knows he is still very normal. This is what must be guarded against very carefully. As always, the speech therapist will assess the patient and plan a treatment programme. However, unlike the other speech problems in which the programme can be carried out jointly between therapist, relatives and nurses, the therapist may feel that if the problem is sufficiently severe he may need treatment by the expert all the time. Therefore, after assessment, she may advise the relatives on the patient's level of understanding and how best to communicate with him, as has been previously described, but she may wish to carry out all the direct therapy herself. A receptive dysphasia is a very complex problem and in the early days is really best handled by the expert alone.

When the speech therapist has made the patient aware of his problems, and he knows what he must do to facilitate better language comprehension, then she may wish to enlist the help of others.

Always with a receptive problem, the starting point is *input*. Until this problem has been dealt with there can be no meaningful *output*. Were the problem to be approached the other way round and the *output* level tackled first, you could perhaps get the patient to name words after you quite happily. For example, you might teach him to say 'bed', but he would not be able to apply it in context if he felt tired. He would merely be repeating it parrot fashion. Also, to start work at this level would mean that you were rewarding with praise a response which you should really be inhibiting.

If the patient is not understanding you, he is probably not understanding himself, he may be unable to sequence his thoughts into some logical pattern. Therefore, the speech therapist will train him to listen carefully to what is said to him, process this in his mind, and produce the appropriate response. This is the response which must be strongly rewarded with praise, not the utterance, albeit correct, of an inappropriately used word.

In fact, the speech therapist will spend very little time on the patient's speech output in these early days. Her main concern will be to get him to begin listening and comprehending. The response for which she is aiming is normally a gestural one in that she will give him a simple command: e.g. 'Pick up the pen!' He will have to listen carefully, interpret the message and perform the appropriate action, thus showing that he has comprehended. She may also work on reading, this also being an input task. This does not mean repeating after you the word which is written. At this stage of therapy this would only be a meaningless response. But, matching the appropriate written word to an object or picture which it describes. Work must therefore be done intensively on *input*, because when his mind has been dealt with he may be able to use the words which he has in a meaningful way.

One of the main *output* problems with receptive dysphasics is that, where they have to be taught to listen to you, they likewise have to be taught to listen to themselves. They may believe that they are communicating with you and may not realise that they are producing jargon. Again, this is something that they must be made aware of. They have to be encouraged to listen to their own speech, check their own output and realise when they are producing jargon.

From childhood we have been able to comprehend and speak automatically not really consciously listening to either the input or the output. After a stroke as described here this is no longer automatic, and listening must be taught as a new skill. However, once that skill has been learned and the patient realises that sometimes he doesn't understand and doesn't speak logically, then he is on the road to recovery. Perhaps his language will never return completely, but, with the help of the speech therapist and the care of the family, he can hopefully reach a level of communication which is adequate for his everyday needs and which reduces frustration.

b. *Expressive dysphasia*

With this problem, language and communication are again greatly reduced. Reading, writing and speaking are affected but comprehension for the greater part is intact. Hence, the patient can understand what is being said, is generally able to form a logical response in his own mind, but cannot find the correct words to put his response into speech.

There are several ways in which this problem presents itself. In the most severe form, the patient may be virtually speechless, perhaps only able to say 'yes' and 'no', and these may be used, as is often the case with all dysphasias, inconsistently and inappropriately. The patient may also have a recurrent utterance, i.e. he may continue to say the same meaningless phrase, e.g. 'comes and been' every time he attempts speech. Patients with not quite so much damage may be able to communicate in single words and short phrases, their ability to produce grammatical sentences having been reduced. Finally, in its less severe form, the patient may be able to speak almost normally, but may occasionally have difficulty in finding the words he wants.

Word-finding difficulty is common to all patients with an expressive dysphasia; it is as if their mind momentarily goes blank and they have really to think and search to find the words. The other problem for these patients is that when they produce a word it may be the wrong one. For example, they may mean to say 'television' but instead produce 'chair'. Or, if they do say 'television', which may be the correct response, all subsequent responses may be 'television' — the needle has a habit of getting stuck! This can be tremendously frustrating because the patient with the purely expressive problem, as you would expect, has a greater ability to hear himself than the receptively damaged patient. Thus, his own responses are often as frustrating to him as they are to the listener.

As already stressed, the problem affects language as a whole, therefore, as with speech, his reading and writing will also be affected to a greater or lesser extent. The patient may be able to read and comprehend simple words, or, he may be able to read the newspaper headlines and possibly the television programme. If he is not so severely damaged, he may manage to read and comprehend a short paragraph or newspaper article. Writing, as this is an output task, is always much poorer than reading and you will find that writing ability generally falls far short of reading comprehension.

When assessing these patients, the speech therapist is going to look firstly at comprehension. Although this is an expressive dysphasia, there are often comprehension problems in the early days. These are not necessarily due to language loss, but to fatigue and general exhaustion. Having a stroke takes a tremendous amount out of a person, and he may quite simply be far too tired to concentrate on what is being said. Therefore, the speech therapist must assess how long he can concentrate for. She may even decide that five or ten minutes language stimulation is all that he can cope with at any one time. This assessment of therapy time is something which applies to all the communication problems, not just the expressive one. Hopefully, as he gets stronger, his tolerance to therapy will improve.

Once the speech therapist has assessed any input problem, she will look at the main problem which in this case is output. She will want to know the exact level at which the patient's language breaks down. How much speech does he have? If there is no propositional (self-elicited or meaningful) speech, can he be stimulated to produce it? Is he communicating with a few words? Is he using words or sentences? When she has found the breakdown level, she will want to look at it in detail. What words is he producing? How often does he have difficulty in finding a word? How often does he find the wrong word by mistake? If he is producing sentences, at which level does his grammar break down? Is he using mainly phrases or sentences? Is he using prepositions, tenses etc. correctly? The therapist will also test reading comprehension. She must know at which level (words, sentences or paragraphs) reading comprehension fails. Lastly she will assess meaningful writing; however, as this is an output task, it will probably not be beyond the one word stage — at most — initially.

With these questions answered, the treatment programme is started at the appropriate breakdown level and follows a normal developmental pattern from there on, working on speaking, reading and writing exercises. As with a receptive dysphasic, the aim is not to get the patient to produce words which are meaningless, but to produce good propositional speech. This is achieved by language stimulation. For example, you would not say to the patient: 'Chair . . . you say it . . . chair!' This is because, as with the receptive dysphasic, you would perhaps get a meaningless, parroted response. It is therefore better to stimulate him by visual and auditory means to produce the correct response. So, the correct way to elicit the word chair would be to say: 'Chair, you sit on a . . .' and, hopefully, the patient would say the word, the brain having received the correct stimulus. You are giving him a cue and this is the best way to help his word finding difficulty.

General communication with these patients is easier, because, unlike the receptive dysphasics, their own thought processes etc. are relatively intact. They know what they want, and by process of elimination, pointing, gesture and/or use of single words, they are often able to express their needs. So, on a basic day-to-day level, it is less frustrating. However, their main frustration arises from the fact that they are aware of what is going on around them. They are listening to conversation and, if involved in a conversation, may want to add a point, contradict what is being said, or crack a joke. Imagine the feelings of an expressive dysphasic patient if he opens his mouth to make a joke and either nothing or meaningless words result. People immediately try and help with what he is wanting to say but it's not funny any more. Or, imagine the immense frustration of having to listen to a conversation with which you disagree violently, and being unable to state your point of view, or indeed, due to paralysis, being unable to get up and walk away from the source of frustration.

Therefore, with an expressive dysphasic patient (indeed all patients with problems of communication) it is essential that you are not only sensitive to a patient's everyday needs, but also to his emotional needs. The best help can sometimes be to imagine yourself in his position, and thereby sharpen your own sensitivity to his communicative needs.

Dyspraxia

This problem generally occurs along with *dysphasia*, either receptive or expressive. It is a complex problem and one which can be difficult to describe. It may even affect the whole body, limbs as well as mouth. However, for the sake of clarity, this section will be coupled with an expressive dysphasia.

Dyspraxia is the term used for difficulty in performing voluntary movements. This is a difficulty in movement performance because of damage to sensory and motor areas of the brain. The word comes from the Greek *praxia*, doing. An understanding of this problem is essential if an intelligent approach is to be made to rehabilitation. Where it concerns the body as a whole it may result in failure to draw coherently, failure to deal effectively with or manipulate objects and failure to integrate acts into sequence. The only way to tackle the problem from a physical point of view is to follow the lines already described. Go right back to the beginning and work right through the infant patterns of motor and sensory development, remembering that a successful outcome may take many weeks (or even months) of treatment. Where it occurs in the area of speech extra help will be needed. It may often go undiagnosed and unnoticed but, in this case, will lead to failure in speech rehabilitation. Therefore, another simple example will be given here as an aid to understanding:

If you ask the patient to stick out his tongue, a receptive dysphasic may not do it because he does not understand the command and a dysarthric may not do it because his muscles are too weak. A *dyspraxic patient* would:

a. understand the command and
b. attempt to perform the movement, but somewhere between comprehending and performing there is a breakdown, and instead of the

tongue coming out it may go to the back of his mouth, or he may say 'pa' or 'm' or make some other movement of his mouth. He has clearly understood but his mouth will not do what he wants it to.

The assessment of this difficulty is really only possible by the speech thera- pist as it is very similar in appearance as an expressive dysphasia and the defining line is not always clear. There is generally a language loss with this problem in that the patient may have a moderate expressive dysphasia, but his communication difficulty may be severe because of the dyspraxia. Part of his problem will be due to word finding difficulty, i.e. the word he wants does not come readily to mind and he really has to search for it. However, it may also be partly due to the dyspraxia, i.e. he does find the correct word in his brain, knows what he wants to say, tries to say it, but the brain does not co-ordinate with the tongue and the lips and the wrong sound comes out.

So, as you can see, the dyspraxic patient, like the dysphasic, may be producing wrong sounds or words and may also have a recurrent utterance, but the neurological reasons are very different.

As previously stated, this problem is generally found with dysphasia. Therefore the patient's reading and writing are affected. His reading level may be slightly higher because there is probably less language loss than with a pure expressive dysphasia. However, this is not the case with writing. Again, because of language loss, but also because (as with the mouth) the brain may not be co- ordinating with the motor performance (this time the arm), writing may be equally poor. Therefore, to all intents and purposes, these two problems (dysphasia and dyspraxia) are very similar in the picture which they represent.

When the speech therapist has diagnosed a dyspraxia, the treatment would probably have a dual purpose. She would treat the dysphasia as described and she would also give exercises to help improve the co-ordi- nation of the lips, tongue etc. Relaxation is also an important factor; therapy sessions should be as stress free as possible because the more tense these patients become the harder it is for them to co-ordinate. Family and nurses can help by offering the same kind of treatment they should give to the patient with expressive dysphasia. The patient can understand so speak to him normally, stimulate his responses but don't get him to repeat unless the speech therapist specially asks for this as part of the treatment programme.

In a very few cases, it is possible to find an almost pure dyspraxia, i.e. language involvement is minimal. These patients may therefore still be able to read books and may perhaps be able to write single propositional words, which they can use as a dual means of communication along with whatever speech they have. However this is not a very common disorder, and is best described to you by the speech therapist who diagnoses it.

Dysarthria

With this problem, as previously stated, there is no language loss. Generally speaking, the patient can read and write, he knows or understands what you are saying and in return he will speak in perfectly logical, well-formed sentences which, however, due to muscle weakness, are often barely intelligible.

Characteristically, speech is slow, slurred, monotonous and often nasal. This is due to weakness of the lips, tongue and soft palate. Hence, you may also find that the patient has difficulty in eating and is prone to drooling, which is a tremendous social handicap, and which can further lead to his feeling of isolation and inadequacy.

When the speech therapist assesses the dysarthric patient she is going to look firstly at the sounds he is making. She must find out the following:

1. What sounds can he make?
2. What sounds can he approximate?
3. What sounds are lost?

She will then find out if his breathing pattern is accurate for speech — does he have enough breath to raise his voice, or to say a sentence? This leads to other questions. For example, at what pace does he speak, is it abnormally fast or slow? Is his speech pretty monotonous, or is he managing some intonation to colour it? In other words, does he produce the normal rise and fall of the voice when speaking?

Once these questions have all been answered, the speech therapist will decide upon a treatment programme which, as always, can be carried out by nurses and/or relaltives as advised by her.

Treatment would involve exercises to improve movement in the lips, tongue and palate and here the physiotherapist can often give her expert advice. Together she and the speech therapist may devise a suitable scheme of exercises that will help to overcome the problem. A small block of *wet* ice may be used to good effect to massage affected facial muscles. For ice treatment and for exercise the physiotherapist thinks in terms of muscle direction and she may use her fingers or a wooden spatula to give any desired assistance or resistance to any movement. The exercises offered jointly by the speech therapist and the physiotherapist may include some, or all, of the following suggestions. Exercises may be given unilaterally or bilaterally (or both) and, if necessary, will include eyebrows, eyes, nose and mouth. The therapist may use her fingers and thumbs to depress the eyebrows and then ask her patient to raise them, giving assistance or resistance as necessary. He may be asked to screw up his eyes while she gives resistance to the movement, to sniff against mild resistance given when she closes his nostrils with finger and thumb, and to smile and then to purse his lips with assistance and against resistance. He may be asked to suck against resistance offered by two wooden spatulas which are held inside his mouth with a mild lateral pull to give a wide grin. The tongue will be exercised against resistance offered by the wooden spatula and jaw movements are practised. The help of a mirror for facial exercises may be necessary. Breathing exercises will be given, and exercises to improve the accuracy of the speech sounds. Any intonation exercises given to reduce the monotony of the patient's speech will include phrasing exercises. Using short phrases instead of long sentences obviously improves the clarity. Likewise, reminding the patient to speak slowly and clearly. Therapy for the dysarthric patient can therefore be undertaken jointly by the speech therapist and the physiotherapist.

When you have been advised about exercises, it is essential that they are practised regularly every day. With a little effort, speech can become more intelligible and general quality of voice will improve and become more pleasant.

With some patients, there may be drooling and difficulty in swallowing food. Here, the speech therapist may be able to demonstrate some techniques which can be employed to reduce the problem. However, one thing to remember is that swallowing saliva may no longer be automatic.

If there is a facial paralysis and weakness of the muscles of the mouth, the swallowing reflex may be reduced and the patient may be unaware of saliva gathering in his mouth. So, having someone to remind him that he needs to swallow is often more helpful than giving him a handkerchief to wipe his mouth. He can often be taught to remember to swallow. The next point applies to all stroke patients with communication problems, but especially to those who are dysarthric. *Dentures* and *hearing-aids* must be examined. Always, after a stroke, have the hearing-aid checked to ensure that it is working efficiently, and indeed it may be advisable to have the hearing re-tested. Likewise, consult the dentist. Find out if the existing dentures still fit or would they benefit from a re-line to make them better fitting. Perhaps the patient may require a complete new set. Make sure that maximum benefit is being received from these aids.

Lastly, as there is generally no language involvement, the dysarthric patient may still be able to write. However, in a few patients writing may be difficult for various reasons and some retraining by the speech therapist may be necessary. Writing can often be used along with speech as a dual means of communication, and some severely dysarthric patients may find writing to be a necessary alternative.

Summing-up

1. Remember the golden rule which has been stressed throughout this whole section: speak to the patient as you would speak to any normal intelligent adult.
2. Remember that with the dysphasic patient, reading and writing are also affected. Therefore, *never* give a patient a paper and pencil and

ask him to write down what he is trying to say. This only causes frustration and depression: remember it is language as a whole which is affected.

3. Likewise, don't give him the usual load of paperbacks and magazines which are so much a part of hospital visiting. In the early days he may become even more depressed when he realises that his reading ability is greatly reduced. However, as he becomes stronger and more able to cope with his disability it is advisable to restart his daily paper and favourite magazine. Even if he can only read the headlines and look at the pictures, he is becoming reorientated and will benefit from the language stimulation. At this stage you can also read out short articles to the patient, letting him follow the words with you.

4. Arithmetic is also generally affected. So, don't trust him to pay the milkman unless you leave the exact money!

5. For all speech damaged patients, dysarthric, dyspraxic and dysphasic, another essential rule applies: *never* stop and talk unless you have time to listen. If you are busy just wave or shout a cheery 'hallo!' Communication with these patients is slow and it is obviously more frustrating for them if you stop to chat briefly and have to leave without finding out what they are saying. Therefore, it is important that you strike a happy balance between the cheerful wave and 'hallo', and being able to sit down at length for a chat.

6. Communication charts must be mentioned. There are two or three types available. These are charts with pictures of articles the patient may need, e.g. toilet, spectacles etc. We have found that these are of little value to a dysphasic patient, and are only really of any use with the dysarthric patient. The dysphasic patient may be unable to select the appropriate picture due to damaged mental processing, or, as these patients often have visual problems, they may be unable to see or recognise the pictures due to an excess of visual stimulus. Therefore, these charts, if used inappropriately, can be a further source of frustration and so the advise of the therapist should be sought before introducing them.

7. Positioning is also very important during speech therapy (indeed as it must be twenty-four hours a day following a stroke). The patient should be positioned carefully in the correct chair with a table at a suitable working height as already described. Speech therapy requires tremendous concentration from the patient and if spasticity and pain develop, his power of concentration will be reduced. Therefore, correct positioning before commencing treatment is essential.

8. Finally, we purposely have not included any specific exercises for the dysphasic and dyspraxic patients because *this is virtually impossible to do* without knowing the individual patient and his problem. The differential diagnosis between dyspraxia and receptive and expressive dysphasia is a job for the speech therapist, who, having assessed, will

advise you on exercises which will be appropriate to the patient. To perform 'speech exercises' with a patient who has not been profesionally assessed is of little value and can, if wrongly administered, lead yet again to frustration. There should be a speech therapist in your area; however, if you cannot contact one, the general secretary at the following address will be able to put you in touch with the nearest available speech therapist:

College of Speech Therapists, Harold Poster House, 6 Lechmere Road, London NW2 5BU.

5

Progress through exercise

As has already been said, rehabilitation means progress, through exercise, to the maximum degree of physical and psychological independence of which a patient is capable.

A series of diagrams will now be given to show the main exercise positions used by the physiotherapist as she continues her rehabilitation programme for the stroke patient. The brief notes that accompany each diagram are aimed at better understanding. Many of the exercises may be used for home care and, indeed, frequently the stroke patient will carry out many of his own exercises but, in severe disability, it is hoped that a physiotherapist may have been involved from the beginning. With early and careful handling and training by the expert, difficulties that would later lead to severe and irreversible disability may be avoided.

As exercise progresses, care must continue to be taken to make sure that the patient continues to live *at all times in the pattern*. This, by now, will be understood to mean sleeping, sitting and standing in the correct way and weight-bearing through a correctly positioned base at all times. All activities will be carried out as far as possible with the patient maintaining correct practices. For example, watching television is often a favourite convalescent activity. It does not make too great a demand on a tired body and severe fatigue is often a symptom in the early days. But, for this simple activity, it is urgently necessary for the patient to be seated correctly. His affected leg is bent to 90° at the hip and knee and the foot is positioned on the floor (as indicated in Fig. 43) so that the hip does not roll into external rotation. At the same time, the patient's affected arm is correctly supported (as indicated in Fig. 30). He leans on his forearm, remembering that his hand must not stray across the red line. The television set is positioned so that he rotates slightly towards his affected side to watch the screen, thus helping to support his body weight correctly from elbow to shoulder.

It will also be understood that all patients do not necessarily follow an identical exercise programme. The expert — be this the doctor, or the therapist with the doctor's backing — will fully understand the patient's tolerance to exercise and will advise treatment accordingly. The programme should always be related to the patient's age and/or other physical disabilities.

Weight-bearing over the correctly positioned base and careful maintenance of inhibiting patterns is of prime importance and exercises may often be adapted or modified to suit the individual. Where any other medical condition makes full rehabilitation an impractical goal, the expert may advise a quick return to walking by using a walking-aid as support on the sound side of the body so that the patient learns to compensate for his disability solely by the use of his sound side. In this case, it must be accepted that he will never again have full and functional use of the affected side of his body. To promise anything else is to make a promise that cannot be kept. However, even in this case, correct positioning in lying and sitting may help to prevent the onset of the crippling disability of excessive spasticity. Whatever the circumstances, a calliper that supports the affected knee and leads to quicker walking will inevitably give pressure (or weight-bearing) on the front part of the foot (a wrongly positioned base). This will lead to a build-up of spasticity and *is not generally advisable*.

The physiotherapist aims all the time at helping her patient to reach the maximum independence of which he is capable and, to do this, he must be taught to use both sides of his body. Because of the special difficulties that are encountered when handling the stroke patient, and the need to maintain round-the-clock positioning, she welcomes all the help that can be given by her patient's family and friends and all who have any dealings with him. As each patient is different (no two stroke patients picked at random will present exactly the same symptoms) the physiotherapist will tailor her treatment programme to fit the individual. *But,* the need for diligent positioning does not alter and gives a common ground for a basic treatment pattern. The following exercise positions fit the basic pattern and are given here to assist the reader towards the basic understanding that is necessary if the home team is to assist in the rehabilitation programme. And, if the patient is cared for at home, it is urgently necessary for the home team to play a correctly supporting role.

Figure 44 is included as a reminder that the infant's pattern of sensory and motor development continues to be related to stroke care. The rehabilitation programme continues to follow this sequence; rolling leads to propping, propping to crawling, and crawling to walking.

At all times, special care should be taken by all who deal with the patient to hold fast to the following points:

1. You must help him to maintain correct positioning.
2. Correct positioning must include his furniture so that he is encouraged to assist recovery by working across mid-line from the sound side of his body to the affected side. *Approach him from his affected side.*
3. All movement takes place within the recovery pattern, i.e. into the inhibiting pattern and away from the spasticity pattern.
4. The arm will be mobilised into external rotation.
5. The leg will be mobilised into internal rotation.

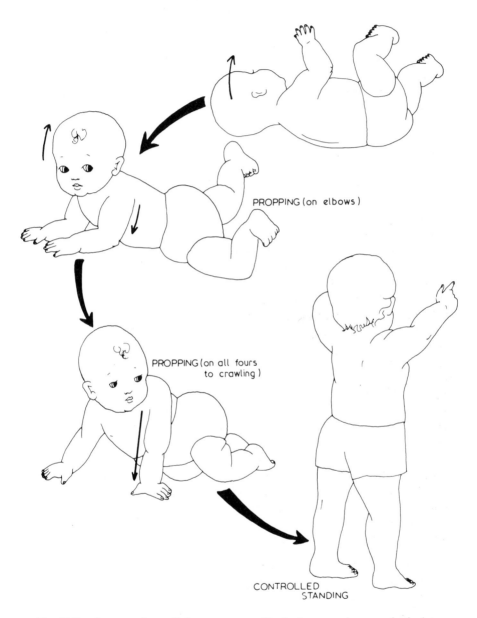

PROPPING (on elbows)

PROPPING (on all fours
to crawling)

CONTROLLED
STANDING

Fig. 44 Development of controlled movement — rolling leads to propping, propping leads to crawling, crawling leads to walking.

6. Weight-bearing will be used as much as possible but you must make sure that this includes *correct positioning of the standing base*.

Before going any further, note that the exercises already described must be continued. You must make sure that you have got the arm position of external rotation correct. (Consult Fig. 16.)

Note. The positions in which the patient must be stabilised, or must attain perfect balance, will be marked in the text with a star (★). They are placed in the order they should follow and it is important not to leave out any single progression.

Figure 45: Getting down on to the floor

This will not be attempted until the previous exercises have been mastered and the patient has reached a fair degree of independence as described. With the patient standing (hands clasped, palms touching) the helper may stand behind him with her hands under his arms and lower him backwards to the floor. Or the method illustrated may be used. But, whatever method is used, it will undoubtedly need the help of two people to get the patient up off the floor in the early days. Therefore, for some patients at this stage, it may be necessary to continue exercises on the bed and leave floor exercise until later.

As soon as possible (as illustrated) a solid piece of furniture that makes a suitable seat also serves as a second helper. Also as illustrated, the handshake grasp given by the helper to the patient's affected arm maintains the necessary external rotation of his shoulder and leaves her second hand free to support his elbow.

A bed mattress placed on the floor may be used in the early days to give adequate padding because exercises will be freely interspersed with rest periods using careful positioning. As soon as the patient begins rolling to propping the mattress may be used crosswise to support his head and trunk and his feet may rest on the floor. Many patients find a suitably warm room with a carpeted floor quite adequate for the exercise session. In this case use pillow support for resting positions.

As the helper, once your patient is safely on the floor, make sure you do not omit the very necessary shoulder movements shown in Figures 16, 17 and 18. It is important to note that if early shoulder movements give pain you may look for two possible causes:

1. The patient is not being nursed with due care and correct positioning is not being maintained.

2. The arm is not being held in the correct inhibiting pattern and the correct pattern is not being maintained during movement.

It is suggested you go back and check your positioning from the beginning.

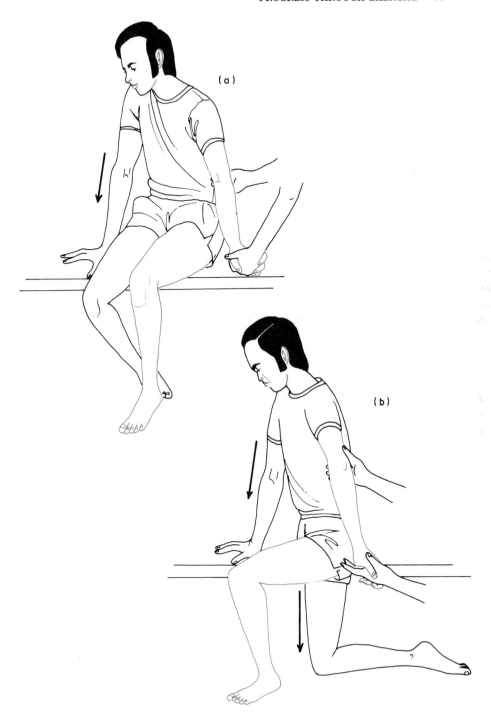

Fig. 45 (**a** & **b**) Getting down onto the floor from stool

Figure 46*: Rolling to the affected side (Lying on the affected side)

This exercise ought to have been established in bed but it is much easier to do on the floor. The patient has room to move with no fear of falling. He is taught to use the handclasp position as illustrated, with his palms touching, his elbows straight and his hands held at, or above, shoulder level. This makes sure that the shoulder is maintained in the required position. Teach him to lead the movement with his eyes and rotate his head to the side to which he is turning. Shoulder rotation follows as he leads on round with his hands. Trunk rotation, legs following, is usually an automatic follow up and very soon needs little or no outside assistance. As shown in the illustration, this is a very good resting position because the shoulder is well placed forwards in external rotation and has not been allowed to become trapped under the body. While resting in this position, the hip is well placed if it is straight instead of bent. As the patient has to spend so much time with the hip bent in the recovery (or inhibiting) pattern there is a danger of stiffness developing, so this position is better. This diagram illustrates the one position where the hip may safely be left in extension for lengthy resting periods. If this point is neglected, the patient may later not be able to get his hip straight enough for good walking. Rolling must be established. Recovery starts first in the muscles of the trunk. He must learn to balance firmly on his affected side.

Figure 47*: Rolling to the sound side (Lying on the sound side)

As has already been said, initially this movement may give trouble but it must be mastered. *Make* your patient use his eyes by standing, or kneeling, on the side to which he is turning and attract his attention by clapping your hands. As he turns to look at you give him a loud, clear command: 'Come on, reach your hands round to me!' Hold out a hand to meet his hands and assist the turn with your other hand. Once again, this is a very good resting position and resting in a good position is thoroughly therapeutic. During the turn, the affected knee rolls over in front of the sound knee (if not, help to place it there) and the affected hip automatically turns well into the correct pattern of internal rotation. Frequent resting in this position will do much to prevent the tight externally rotated hip that will develop with build-up of spasticity in the neglected patient. If this is allowed to happen, the resulting stiff, badly-positioned hip will make a normal walking pattern quite impossible. Balance is again established.

The patient must be taught to maintain the side lying positions. In the words of the physiotherapist, *he must be stabilised in side lying*. This is done by asking him to 'hold' a position against gentle pressure offered by the helper, **but**, when this pressure is given, muscle tone will increase and so it is of vital importance always to make sure that his whole body is positioned and 'holding' in the complete inhibiting pattern. Otherwise the increased tone *will increase spasticity*.

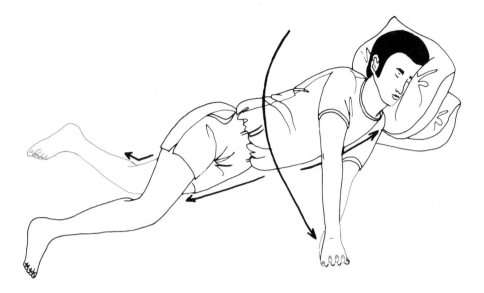

Fig. 46 Rolling to the affected side

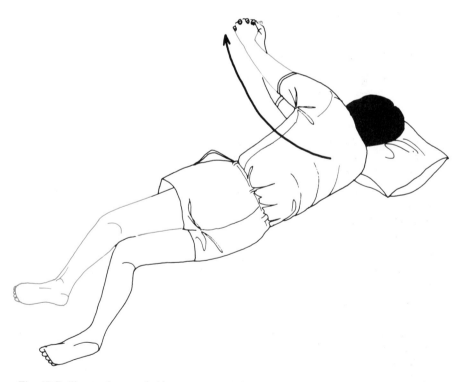

Fig. 47 Rolling to the sound side

These are the first two balancing positions which *must be taught*. The other necessary positions will follow.

Figure 48*: Rolling to propping on the affected elbow (Elbow propping)

Again, this exercise ought to have been established in bed. If so, it will be carried out readily on the floor. The floor, even where a mattress is used, gives a much firmer support. This makes exercise positions much easier to achieve. Where rolling to propping is established early and correctly, there is a fair chance of a return to reasonable arm function. It is one of the necessary steps to recovery that must not be omitted, remembering that recovery proceeds from trunk to shoulder. You can help the patient to reach the required position by placing his affected elbow out to the side of his body and holding it in place with one of your hands while you use your other hand to take his sound hand firmly in a handshake grasp. With a cross pull, assist him forwards and sideways into position. When he has learnt to balance on the correctly positioned elbow, and has been stabilised in this position, he may spend some time maintaining it while, for example, he turns the pages of a magazine, drinks a cup of tea which has been carefully placed in position, or plays a game of solitaire.

Figure 49: Back lying hip rolling

Remembering that recovery proceeds from trunk to hip, this is an important exercise because it is essential to establish early hip control. Give assistance and help your patient to do slow rhythmical knee rolling from side to side, progressing to unassisted movement. Later you can make him work a little harder by altering the assistance given to slight resistance. Aim at teaching him to progress to stretching the sound leg out straight and, keeping the affected knee bent, repeat the exercise with the one leg until a slow, controlled movement is possible. Support the leg in the bent position where necessary so that it is not allowed to straighten out into the spasticity pattern. For resting periods both knees will be bent up and the knees will point to the ceiling (or towards the sound side) — thus maintaining the recovery pattern. Tap firmly on the inside of the affected knee as a reminder if the patient forgets his positioning during resting and allows the knee to drift outwards so that the hip is badly positioned in external rotation. There is always a tendency to drift into the pattern of spasticity. The following notes on 'bridging' will be helpful in this case.

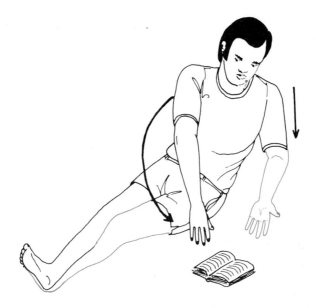

Fig. 48 Rolling to propping on the elbow

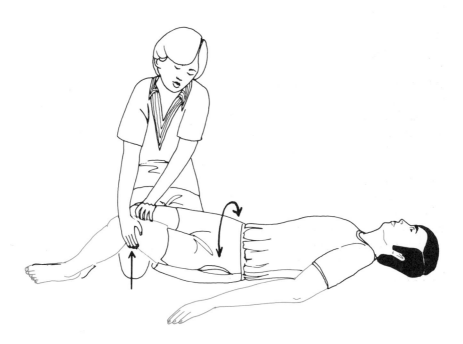

Fig. 49 Back lying hip rolling

Figure 50*: Bridging (The bridging starting position)

A repeat of Figure 15 and this exercise *must* have been established in bed. Its importance has already been stressed — refer to the text on Figure 15. Remember, where the patient has difficulty in maintaining the position, teach him to hold a book between his knees. At first he may need assistance to hold the book in position, or he may only succeed in holding it for a few seconds before the affected knee falls away as the leg drifts into the forbidden spasticity pattern of external rotation of the hip. But he will quickly learn to hold it for much longer periods and soon will no longer need the book. You may find it necessary to support the affected leg in the correct position while the patient 'bridges' by lifting both buttocks off the floor. Very soon you should be able to reinforce the exercise by giving a little pressure as indicated by the arrows.

Rolling should now be established. This means the patient rolls over on to his face; rolling over and over across the floor will follow. His hands *must* be clasped with palms touching, and held at or above shoulder level to maintain correct shoulder positioning. A wrongly positioned shoulder which is trapped under the body during rolling will give nothing but trouble and intense pain. Rolling to the sound side may continue to need encouragement from you. Remember to keep on the side to which the patient is rolling.

Figure 51*: Rolling to elbow propping (both elbows)

Look at Figure 44 and note how the infant rolls to elbow propping. Lifting his head backwards helps to stabilise his arms and bend his knees. In the early days place a pillow under the patient's shins to prevent full leg extension while you concentrate on helping your patient to prop correctly over both forearms. The mirror helps the necessary neck extension. Stabilise in this position using supporting pressure laterally on his shoulders. If he sags to one side, increase your pressure on the opposite shoulder so that he pushes up into the required position. As soon as forearm propping is fully stabilised, as illustrated, the leg exercise may be given. At first the exercise will be passive. This means that you will move the patient's legs for him. The mirror must be placed so that he can watch the movement. Later in the programme he will help with the movement; much later he will go it alone.

Note. A weak shoulder which is thoroughly stabilised in this position will almost certainly be, or will quickly become, a pain free shoulder. If the elderly patient with stiff lumbar spine (low back), or arthritis or any other condition, fails to establish full rolling and the necessary forward lying with correct arm positioning, the physiotherapist ought to be able to suggest suitable exercise modifications (see Fig. 70).

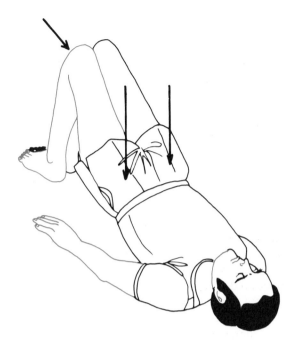

Fig. 50 Bridging

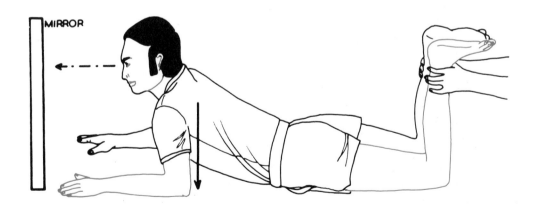

Fig. 51 Rolling to elbow propping

Figure 52: Hip and knee movement

Here, by bending his sound leg and clasping his hands round his sound knee, the patient is actively assisting the physiotherapist. He is using his affected arm in an acceptable position. Also, bending his sound hip helps to initiate movement in the affected hip. The physiotherapist is using a good handgrip. She is separating his toes into the inhibiting pattern and supporting his weak knee. At first the movement is passive. This means that she moves the leg. She is bending and stretching the hip and knee but she does not allow the leg to stretch out fully into the spasticity pattern. Later in the rehabilitation programme she will ask the patient to help her with the movement and, as he gains hip and knee *control*, she will gradually withdraw her support. Then she will teach her patient to hold the leg quite still in space without any support from her in the position illustrated. But this is a much later progression after many more exercise routines have been taught. 'Holding in space' is very difficult — more difficult than movement — and control of the limb is very good by the time the patient is able to do this. Until this kind of control is reached, in the words of the physiotherapist, the limb will not be maintained in space but will drift into the spasticity pattern. Remember, these progressions may take many months to achieve and at no time must the patient be expected to move forward from one progression to the next without first obtaining stability in each position marked with a star (*).

How can the home team best help? You can help by assisting the patient to maintain meticulous positioning at all times and by using the handling that will bring success to each stage he reaches. *He must live in the recovery pattern.*

Figure 53: Hip rolling

This has been included to reinforce the last point and as a reminder that, whatever resistance the helper offers to a movement, the effort made by the patient must not be allowed to lead to unwanted muscle pull in other parts of the body. In other words, as illustrated, the patient is being asked to pull his knee inwards against too strong a resistance offered by the physiotherapist's left hand. Why too strong a resistance? As shown in the diagram, the effort the patient is making to roll his hip inwards against the pressure on his knee is also making him roll his affected shoulder into the spasticity pattern. (See section 6, Figs 95 and 96 for help with this problem.)

The essential rule in stroke rehabilitation is to keep on checking positioning. Where the lower limb is being exercised, check positioning of the upper limb, and vice versa. Do not make a demand the patient is not ready to meet.

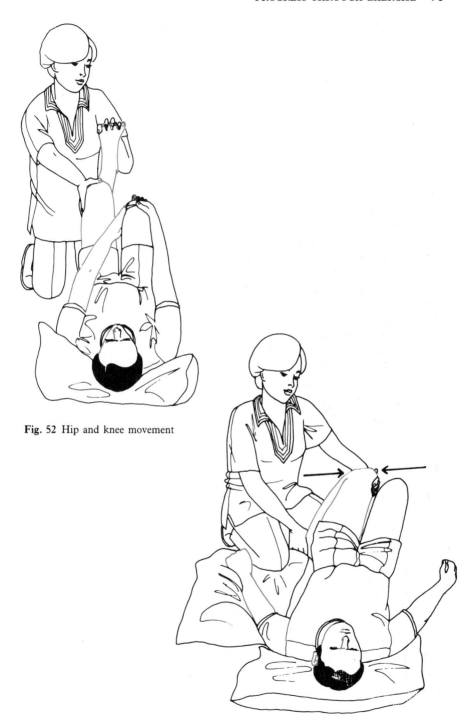

Fig. 52 Hip and knee movement

Fig. 53 Hip rolling

Figure 54: Hand clasp position

Refer now to Figure 4 (p. 14). At no time in the early days of motor control does the infant appear to clasp his hands. The question will be asked, why does the stroke patient spend so much time with hands clasped? There are three main reasons:

1. To help him to live in the recovery pattern. He is maintaining good positioning. Clasped hands separate the fingers and, with thumbs uppermost, prevent the affected shoulder from rolling inwards. Also, he is taught to use the sound hand to help extend the affected elbow and roll the shoulder outwards so that the affected palm faces upwards towards the ceiling.

2. He is frequently unaware of the affected hand and, if this neglect is allowed to continue, he will never use it again. Clasping it with his sound hand brings it into mind and into his mental picture of a complete body.

3. In the hand clasp position he must then be taught to hold his palms together. This will help the fingers to relax and will complete the necessary arm recovery pattern.

In the stages given so far the patient ought to have thoroughly mastered side lying, rolling from side to side, bridging, rolling to prop on the affected elbow, rolling to sit on the edge of the bed and stability in sitting. He will need active assistance in all other movements. Do not expect too much from him. Exercise sessions ought not to be too demanding; remember that resting with good positioning is an integral part of every exercise session. On the other hand, make it possible for him to achieve the required positions by offering correct help. He must not be made to feel helpless because the independence that correct handling would give is being denied.

Figure 55: Resting within the recovery pattern

The elderly patient may need to have frequent resting periods during any exercise session. Any position which the patient finds comfortable may be used *as long as it keeps within the recovery pattern*. Remember that particular care must always be taken to see that the affected hip is not allowed to roll outwards into external rotation and the affected shoulder is not allowed to roll inwards into internal rotation. Both side lying positions already illustrated (Figs 46 and 47) give good resting positions, or lying on the back with both knees bent up (as in Fig. 56) and the affected arm carefully positioned on pillows. In the latter position it helps the recovery pattern if the patient is taught to roll both knees away from the affected side towards the sound side. Supporting pillows must be adequate to maintain good positioning for all resting periods. All patients frequently fall asleep in the early days after onset of the stroke and to sleep within the recovery pattern is a necessary part of any long-term rehabilitation programme.

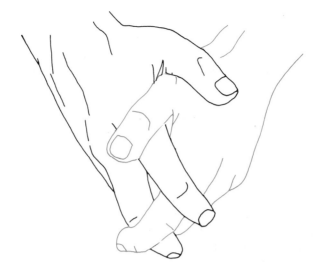

Fig. 54 Hand clasp position

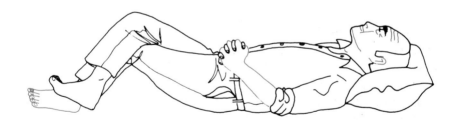

Fig. 55 Resting within the recovery pattern

Figure 56 Crook-lying with book held between knees, hands clasped, double arm raising

This exercise is a progression on all previous exercises because it makes a greater demand on the patient's concentration. It combines the starting position that has been learnt for bridging with one of the vital self-care arm exercises. The patient has to remember to hold the book steady while he moves his arms and his palms must be touching.

Figure 57 Crook-lying, arms rotating from side to side (or upper trunk rolling)

If rolling has been properly taught and mastered, this exercise will not give any trouble. Later it can be combined with arms rotating to one side and legs to the opposite side. All trunk rotation exercises help to reduce spasticity and assist trunk-to-shoulder and trunk-to-hip recovery. You must never forget to pay particular attention to shoulder positioning. As illustrated here, the shoulder is well cared for.

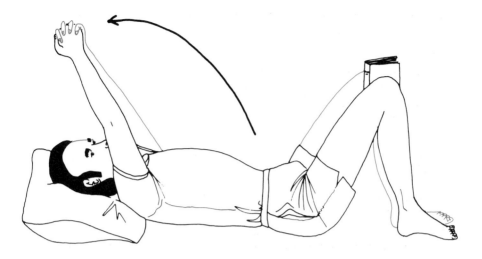

Fig. 56 Crook-lying with book held between knees, hands clasped, double arm raising

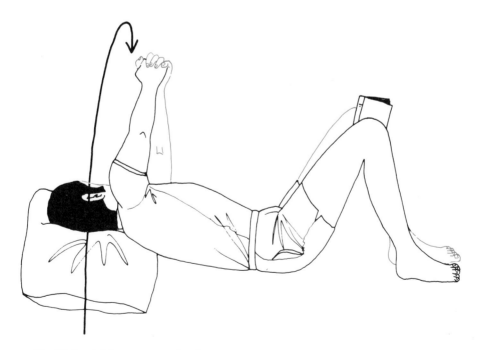

Fig. 57 Crook-lying, arms rotating from side to side (or upper trunk rolling)

Figure 58: Weight-bearing through the heel of the hand

It should by now be fully understood why weight-bearing through the heel of the hand is an essential exercise where maximum arm recovery is to follow. As illustrated, the physiotherapist is supporting her patient's elbow while she interlaces her fingers with his and places the heel of her hand firmly in contact with the heel of his hand. Having taken up this position, they maintain contact and push their hands firmly and gently together as he reaches, or thrusts, forwards with a well-positioned shoulder. Slowly and steadily they build up the pressure they both apply between their hands (as shown by the arrows) and slowly they withdraw it again. The exercise is repeated over and over until the patient is tired.

Figure 59: Shoulder rehabilitation

To assist full external rotation of the shoulder, the physiotherapist will *gently* roll the extended arm from the position illustrated so that the thumb points away from the patient's body and his palm faces round towards her. Emphasis must be placed on the word *gently*. Exercises ought not to be painful. Remember, in the very early days, movements are passive (all movement done by the physiotherapist and none by the patient). As illustrated here, movement has progressed from passive to assisted active with support. Having explained the exercise, the command given to the patient should be short and simple, e.g. 'Watch your hand . . . Now help me to turn your palm toward me . . .' The arrow indicates the movement that is made. The amount of help given by the patient will increase as shoulder function returns. Where there is any risk of shoulder spasticity developing, the patient must not be asked to assist with the turn back to the illustrated starting position. This small movement in the direction of internal rotation will continue to be done passively by the physiotherapist (or by the helper) while active external rotation is encouraged. Support the shoulder so that it is well forward on a pillow before starting the exercise and make sure that the active exercise leads the thumb to point away from the patient's body.

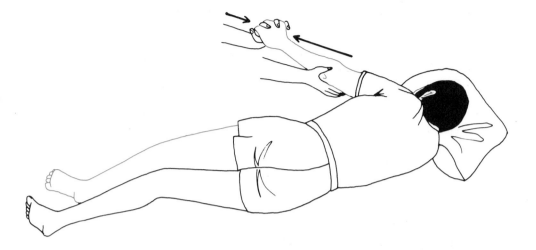

Fig. 58 Weight-bearing through the heel of the hand

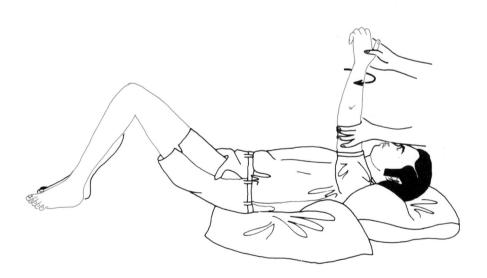

Fig. 59 Shoulder rehabilitation

Figure 60: Side lying, hip straight, assisted knee bending and stretching

This exercise serves a double purpose. (Refer to notes on Fig. 14 concerning his positioning while lying on the affected side.) Once again, by positioning, care is being taken to make sure that the affected hip is not allowed to become stiff and unable to straighten fully. While the patient lies in this position he is well placed for his helper to bend and stretch his affected knee passively. Then she will ask him to think about the movement that is taking place and this leads to the command: 'Help me to bend and stretch your knee.' As rehabilitation progresses he will gradually do more work while she gives less help. It will be understood that voluntary knee movement will not be established until good hip control has been gained. Note that while the leg exercise is given the affected arm has been carefully positioned. Positioning of one limb while the other limb is exercised should by now be established routine and in many cases the patient takes care of this essential point himself.

Figure 61: Side lying, shoulder position maintained while assisted elbow bending and stretching is given (as indicated by arrow)

As in the previous exercise, when this is done passively it helps the patient's brain to remember the movement pattern of bending and stretching the elbow. It must be remembered that the patient must only roll on to a shoulder that is well forward in external rotation. It must not be allowed to become trapped below him in a bad position. It should also be remembered that every roll on to the affected side of the body gives pressure to that side which helps recovery where you have been told the patient has suffered damage to the sensory area of the brain (see Ch. 2).

As illustrated, the physiotherapist or helper has not been included and the patient is resting. To practise the exercise the patient must be alert, with his eyes open, and he should be encouraged to use his eyes to follow the movement of his hand. The same progressions will be made as in the previous exercise. The helper holds the upper arm firmly in position with the shoulder rolled out while she uses her other hand to support his wrist and hand in the position illustrated. He watches the hand as she assists the movement to take the palm of his hand towards his face. Again voluntary elbow movement will not be established until good shoulder control has been gained. Later, she may thread her fingers through his, or use the grip illustrated in Figure 108d, to practise the exercise. This assists the required voluntary movement and keeps the hand away from the spasticity pattern.

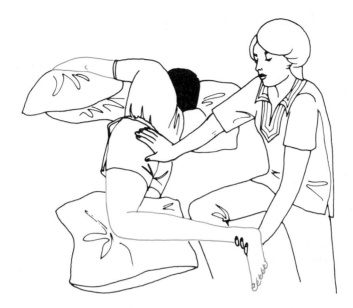

Fig. 60 Side lying, hip straight, assisted knee bending and stretching

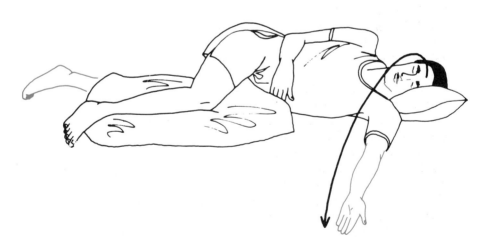

Fig. 61 Side lying, shoulder position maintained while assisted elbow bending and stretching is given (as indicated by arrow)

Figure 62: Shoulder reached well forward, patient pushing (weight-bearing through the heel of the hand)

Where necessary it is hoped that a physiotherapist may be available to give the patient and family instruction for home care.

It does not necessarily follow that the older the patient the longer rehabilitation will take. But, frequently, with the elderly there are more problems in the way of rehabilitation. For example, stiffness from rheumatism may slow up progress and the therapist may have to find a way round such a difficulty. Also, the older brain like the older body may be less resilient. As illustrated here, the therapist is simply giving counter-pressure over the patient's shoulder-blade so that she can exert a stronger force from the heel of his hand to his shoulder. In other words, she is practising the exercise illustrated in Figure 58 and reinforcing the patient's thrust forwards. (Again, this is weight-bearing on a correctly positioned base.) But this exercise ought to be used on young and old alike. The therapist is using her ingenuity to find a way of giving maximum stimulation, the aim being to stimulate postural reflexes as the baby does in crawling on his hands. She should also use this position with these handgrips to assist the movement of rolling the shoulder-blade backwards and forwards round the chest wall. Note that unless meticulous care has been taken at all times with positioning, stiffness and the crippling onset of shoulder pain will have begun. If it is allowed to continue it will effectively put a stop to all worthwhile rehabilitation. What is the answer to this? Go back to the beginning, carefully check all positioning, maintain this correct positioning *24 hours a day* and establish all the shoulder exercises so far given to maintain shoulder mobility.

Figure 63: Arms positioned, shoulder held steady, hip rolling backwards and forwards

All patients ought to establish this exercise but the elderly patient may need more help than the younger man. Here the therapist is helping to hold the shoulders steady in side lying while she assists the hip movement of rolling backwards. She then moves her hand to the back of his hip to assist the movement of rolling the hip forwards. As soon as possible she will move on in her treatment programme to give resistance to the movement of the hip in both directions, backwards and forwards. To roll backwards she places her hand behind the hip and commands: 'Come on, *push* backwards against my hand'. To roll forwards she places her hand as illustrated and asks him to roll the hip forwards against her hand. The affected arm must be carefully positioned and the shoulder held steady so that the fairly strong hip exercise does not make the affected arm pull into the spasticity pattern. She will repeat the exercise on the affected shoulder while she holds the hip steady in side lying.

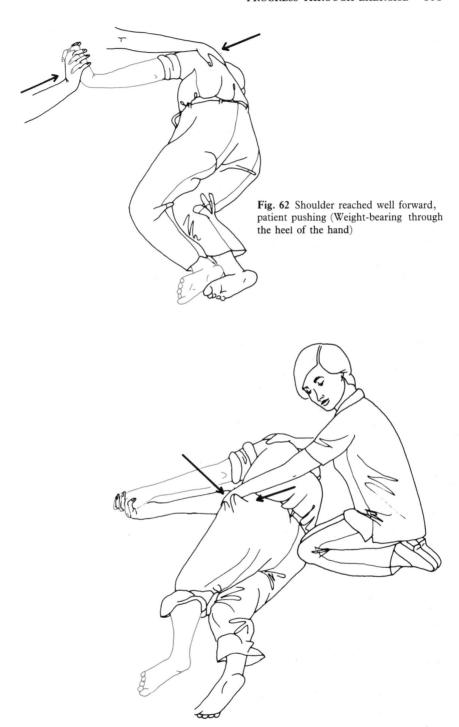

Fig. 62 Shoulder reached well forward, patient pushing (Weight-bearing through the heel of the hand)

Fig. 63 Arms positioned, shoulder held steady, hip rolling backwards and forwards

Figure 64: How to help establish controlled hip bending and stretching

With starting position as for bridging, the patient bends up his sound leg and holds it in position as shown in Figure 64. This serves two purposes. Bending of the sound leg tilts the pelvis (or makes bending of the affected leg easier) and so assists movement of the affected leg. The helper uses one or both of her hands to assist and control the movement. Later she will give graduated and careful resistance to the movement as hip control improves and she will also help the patient to keep the knee in the position illustrated while she removes her supporting hand. For resting periods the legs return to the crook position as used in bridging — never to extension of hips, knees and ankles.

Figure 65: Bridging against resistance

As has already been said, as soon as bridging has been established, the exercise should be reinforced by giving a little downward pressure as indicated by the arrow. This pressure may be given to both hips, or to one side at a time to initiate an active rotation of the pelvis but this is a more advanced exercise. It is harder to achieve. Three separate illustrations on bridging have been included because it is such an important exercise. The patient who cannot bridge will not recover a normal walking gait.

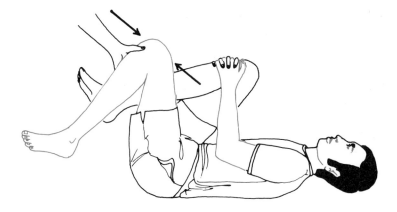

Fig. 64 How to help establish controlled hip bending and stretching

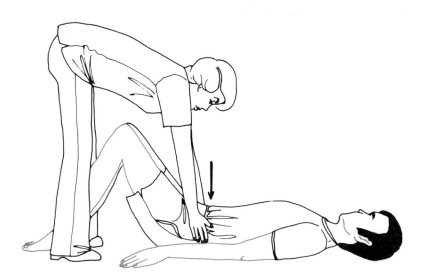

Fig. 65 Bridging against resistance

Figure 66*: Elbow propping

This figure, almost a repeat of Figure 51, has been included as a reminder that rolling practice ought to be included in *every exercise session* and, by now, should have become well-established and ought to be done with comparative ease. Rolling to elbow propping is easy provided the roll over from the back is done with hands clasped and held well above shoulder level. It now ought to be possible to hold the position illustrated without sagging into a poor and less therapeutic posture where weight is not properly distributed from elbow to shoulder. Once again, stabilise the position as previously suggested. Then use the stabilising pressure to increase the shoulder control by teaching the patient to hold quite still against pressure given from any direction. This stabilising pressure may be given to the back of the head (as illustrated), or down through the shoulder, or laterally through either shoulder. It should begin gently, should be increased gradually, and it should be withdrawn gradually. 'Don't let me move you' is a helpful command. The affected leg must be placed with the knee in slight flexion as shown. Note, also, that the forearms must be parallel. This kind of firm stability in elbow propping ought to be established before the next exercise is taught.

Figure 67*: Kneeling with elbow propping

When the patient has been thoroughly stabilised in the previous position, he should be taught to transfer his weight from side to side over alternate forearms. Then he is ready to attempt the more advanced position illustrated in Figure 67, kneeling with elbow propping — or more correctly forearm support. The forearm support has been termed elbow support to emphasise the elbow's position immediately below the shoulder in correct weight-bearing. Initially the physiotherapist may help her patient into position by standing astride his legs (as she did in Fig. 65) and bending to place her hands firmly below his hip bones and lift him upwards and backwards into the kneeling position. As far as he is able, he assists in the movement and draws his forearms backwards to achieve as nearly as possible 90 degrees of bend at his elbows, hips and knees. As indicated by the arrows, he is then stabilised in this position. When he maintains a steady position against reasonable resistance from any direction he is said to be stabilised. Finally, he must be taught to transfer his weight over his affected limbs as a response to lateral pressure — or, pressure given to his affected side.

Note. If the elderly patient finds it difficult to achieve this position a modification is taught, e.g. kneeling with arms positioned on a suitable low table, chair or stool. Here again a physiotherapist may be available to help.

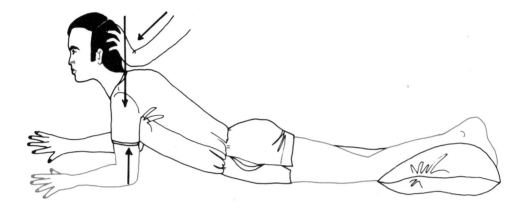

Fig. 66 Elbow propping

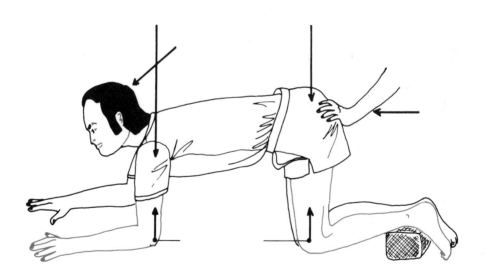

Fig. 67 Kneeling with elbow propping

Figure 68*: Crawling position, thumbs stretched away from other fingers

This thumb position is important because it gives the opportunity of using the arm recovery pattern fully, aiming as far as possible at full hand recovery. This crawling position is the next position in the rehabilitation sequence that the patient must achieve and in which he must attain good balance. A stiff shoulder and wrist can, at this stage, successfully block progress but, if the wrist has been kept fully mobile from the beginning by passive movements, and the shoulder has been diligently cared for by positioning and progressive exercise, there should be no problem.

To begin with, the patient will need assistance to get up from kneeling with elbow propping (Fig. 67) to the crawling position and it will be necessary for the helper to support his weak elbow and shoulder. As already described, he must be stabilised in the position and it may be necessary to support the weak elbow during the next few weeks of treatment while you help him to establish firm balance and to progress to rocking from side to side. He must learn to transfer his weight right over the affected limbs. This will be encouraged if you give a little gentle pressure on the side of his body — *the pressure must be given to his affected side when he is learning to transfer his weight over his affected limbs.* Note that pressure on the sound side to pull him over to the weak side will produce the wrong effect. This will make him pull away from you towards the sound side. He must also learn to rock forwards over his hands. He should be taught to tilt his head backwards and look upwards while you continue to support his elbow with one hand and give a little gentle pressure to the back of his head with the other. This will strengthen the position of the elbow and help to stabilise the position of the affected arm. He should learn to balance in the crawling position while you give gentle pressure to his body from any direction and, at the same time, you continue to support the affected elbow. Take due care of his leg position but, as progress continues, the support to the affected foot (as indicated in Fig. 67) will be withdrawn when the patient is fully stabilised and ready to begin exercises in crawling.

He may learn to stand on his knees (Fig. 69) and begin walking with hands clasped (Fig. 74) before his arm is strong enough for full crawling exercise. The physiotherapist will be able to advise on the rate that progressions ought to be made but be ready to withdraw support from the affected elbow as soon as the patient can maintain the illustrated position alone (Fig. 68).

Figure 69*: Stand kneeling (using mirror)

Again the patient must learn to balance in this position. The illustration once more demonstrates the use of the mirror. Here the physiotherapist is using her hands and her knees to help her patient to maintain the upright

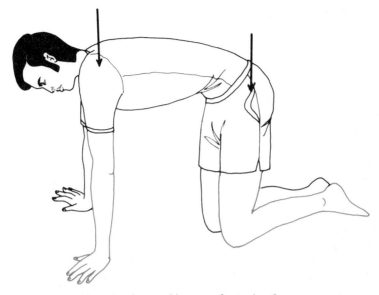

Fig. 68 Crawling position, thumbs stretching away from other fingers

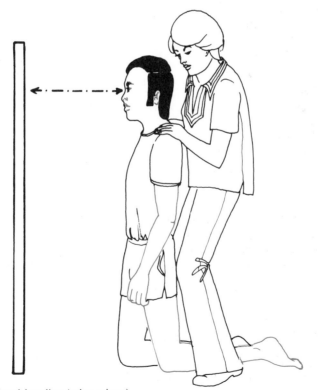

Fig. 69 Stand kneeling (using mirror)

position. With the help of the mirror, the patient's eyes give a necessary extra help towards maintaining the required posture. He will be stabilised by the usual method already described. *To do this his hands ought to be clasped in front with straight elbows* as in Figure 74.

Figure 70: Elbow propping in kneeling

As all the positions marked with a star (*) are thought to be necessary steps in stroke rehabilitation, we are often left with the problem of how best to help the elderly, frail, or otherwise disabled person who has difficulty in following some of the floor routines. Accepting that these positions must be included in any worthwhile treatment plan, it is obvious that a way must be found round any difficulty that is encountered.

Study Figure 70 which is included as a suggested way of treating an elderly patient who finds it impossible to achieve elbow propping as shown in Figure 66. This elderly patient may, for example, have learnt and carefully carried out all the arm, trunk and leg exercises on top of a wide bed. He may have learnt to roll to sitting on the edge of the bed and attained a fair degree of balance in sitting and standing but is defeated by the prospect of rolling round on the floor. Add to this the certain fact that for full therapeutic value exercise sessions ought to be enjoyed. Again, it is necessary to stress that modification in treatment patterns must be introduced. It is not difficult to teach the patient how to transfer from the edge of his bed on to his knees. He uses his sound side and his sound arm to support himself on the bed as he kneels down alongside the bed (consult Fig. 45) and the coffee table is moved into position. He is now in a very good position to begin stabilising in forearm propping exercises and to establish kneeling balance.

Figure 71: Weight transfer over affected forearm

Continuing the rehabilitation of this rather frail elderly man, Figure 71 suggests a way of learning to transfer weight over the affected arm. The cushion has been removed and a brightly coloured stripe struck down the centre of the table top. The reasoning behind this has already been given (consult notes on Fig. 30). If the helper now gives gentle lateral pressure to the affected shoulder (as indicated by the arrow) it will assist the weight transfer over the forearm. It must be gentle pressure; strong pressure will move the arm into the spasticity pattern. If the arm moves, hold it in position and *reduce* the pressure you give. Consult Figure 43c for the position the arm ought to maintain on the table. From this position the patient should be taught to progress to *stand kneeling* as shown in Figure 69. This may be done to advantage with his hands resting on the table. Consult Figure 43a for the position of the hand and remember that elbow support should be given by the helper as long as it is required. Remember

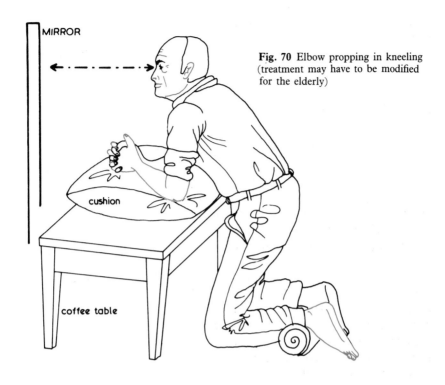

Fig. 70 Elbow propping in kneeling (treatment may have to be modified for the elderly)

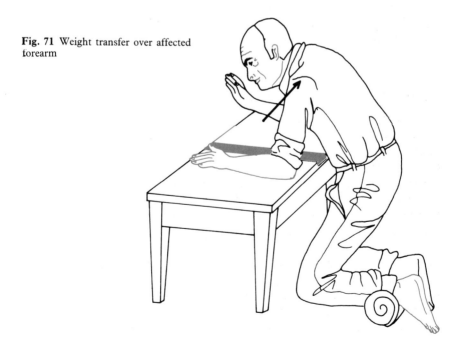

Fig. 71 Weight transfer over affected forearm

also, that if he is taught to tilt his head backwards against gentle pressure it will help to stabilise the arm position.

He ought to be stabilised in all possible propping and kneeling positions.

Figure 72: The elderly patient transfers weight over to his affected side

It may take longer to teach the elderly patient to transfer his weight on to his affected side and extra help in the form of extra support may be needed. But, whatever the age or condition of the patient, this is an exercise he must learn if he is to progress to balanced walking. As illustrated here, the physiotherapist is helping the patient to transfer his weight over his affected side by pushing gently with her hands against his affected hip and his affected shoulder. In response to her pressure — and the command: 'Don't let me push you.' — his body straightens up to stand firmly on both knees and he pushes away from his sound side over on to his affected side.

Even if the patient has been throughly stabilised in stand kneeling (Fig. 69), he frequently needs extra support while he learns to balance over his affected hip and knee. As shown here, the physiotherapist's shoulders are giving this necessary extra support. Perhaps it ought to be stressed once more that where pressure is given by the helper to gain a required response from the patient *it must not become a battle of strength* between the two of them. Pressure must be given gently, must build up slowly until it gains the required response, and must be withdrawn slowly.

If the stroke patient does not learn to transfer his weight properly, he will fail to regain symmetrical control of his body and he will continue to hold his weight over his sound hip with a sagging pelvis while the affected leg remains no more than a rather useless prop.

Figure 73: The elderly patient again using extra support

This illustration shows another way of offering extra support when it is needed. Where necessary the helper places and holds her patient's affected hand (correctly positioned) on top of the stool and supports his elbow. Where he is still learning weight transference', she begins the exercise by making him stand firmly on both of his knees and offering sideways pressure to his affected hip. If both of her hands are occupied in helping him to maintain the correct arm position, she may use her head or her shoulder to give the necessary sideways pressure against his affected shoulder. It is most important that he maintains the arm position correctly and, as he transfers weight over to the affected side, he then stands on a correctly positioned hand.

As a later progression, the patient should be taught to balance and then to lift alternate feet forwards as illustrated.

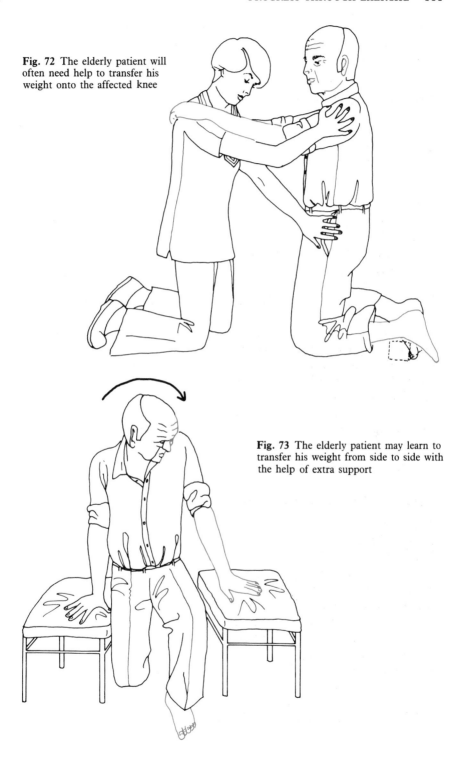

Fig. 72 The elderly patient will often need help to transfer his weight onto the affected knee

Fig. 73 The elderly patient may learn to transfer his weight from side to side with the help of extra support

Figure 74: Knee walking with hands clasped

Knee walking with correct transference of weight from side to side is attempted only after good balance in high kneeling (Fig. 69) has been achieved and the patient has learnt to undertake and control lateral transference of weight over the affected hip. When weight is transferred through the affected hip and knee this frees the sound leg to take a step forward. The patient and the physiotherapist may walk side by side on their knees, practising until the correct movement becomes easy routine. In this case, the physiotherapist will probably hold the patient's affected arm (as illustrated in Fig. 108e) so that he also bears weight through a correctly positioned shoulder each time he transfers over to the affected side. This is also a good arm rehabilitation exercise. The patient may then clasp his hands, palms touching, elbows extended, and begin knee walking alone. This is an exercise which should be carefully and thoroughly mastered because of its importance in the scheme to train symmetrical control of a whole body. In this position, with correct lateral transference of weight, the patient is using his affected hip in the normal pattern of controlled walking without allowing any chance of movement into the extensor spasticity pattern. He is, in fact, performing formal balance walking with weight transference over the affected side. Now he only has to learn to stand up and do this on his feet. Have you noticed that in almost all exercises the physiotherapist approaches her patient from his affected side? This makes an important contribution to successful rehabilitation.

Figure 75*: Crawling position, standing on the affected hand

This is another balancing position which, if possible, ought not to be omitted. It is a very necessary step in regaining good balance and the resulting controlled arm movement which is the aim of all these arm exercises. As might be expected, it closely follows the motor development pattern of the infant (see Fig. 4: 7th month) and, at this stage, may also be attempted using the elbow propping position (Fig. 66). As soon as the patient is thoroughly stabilised in the illustrated position, he should be taught to reach out forwards and sideways in all directions with his sound arm. It often helps to place the mirror in front of him in a suitable position to make him *lean* to reach forward to touch it with his finger-tips without overbalancing.

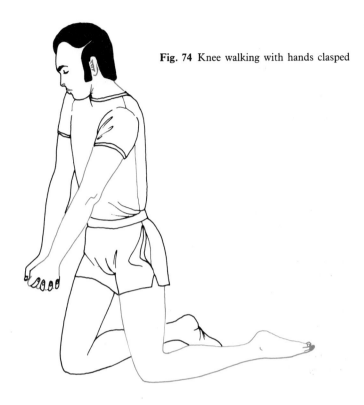

Fig. 74 Knee walking with hands clasped

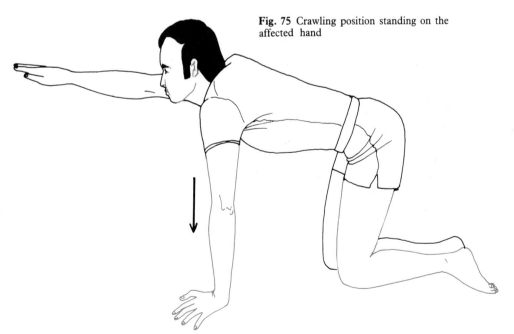

Fig. 75 Crawling position standing on the affected hand

Figure 76: Stand kneeling on a chair

Another modification for the patient who does not find it easy to get down on the floor. Again, this illustration is included as a reminder that a way must be found round any difficulty that stands in the way of good rehabilitation. In this position the patient may be taught good balance in high kneeling and he will then be taught to transfer his weight from side to side as already described. The high-backed chair adds to his feeling of security and his helper is left with both of her hands free to assist him to maintain his balance and to learn the required exercise. Short-cuts may have to be taken but the aim is to establish the whole of the development pattern that leads to controlled posture, where necessary finding a way to do this by the use of skilful modifications. In this case, the help of the physiotherapist is usually necessary and her advice ought to be followed.

To get up onto the chair the patient is correctly supported by his helper on his affected side with the supporting hold illustrated in Figure 108e and is taught to first lift and place his sound knee in the kneeling position on the chair, his affected knee following.

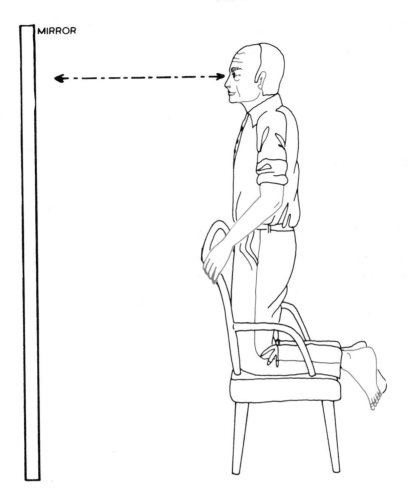

MIRROR

Fig. 76 Stand kneeling on a chair

Figure 77: Learning to balance on alternate knees

This is a progression on the exercise suggested in Figure 73. It is an advanced and difficult exercise and if the patient is asked to attempt it too early in the treatment programme he will fail. It is important to remember that exercise failure can be harmful because it tends to make the patient feel inadequate and helpless. Defeat leads to depression as surely as success leads to a confident and hopeful spirit and a good prospect of useful rehabilitation. So, do not expect your patient to attempt this exercise unless he has successfully mastered all the previous balancing positions.

When establishing this position, the patient clasps his hands (palms touching, elbows straight) to practise lateral transference of his weight. The physiotherapist, or helper, may stand or kneel behind him with her hands placed firmly over both of his hips. She then helps him to transfer his weight over one hip while he lifts the other foot forwards and places it as illustrated. He learns to balance in this position and to change legs and to balance with the other leg placed forwards.

He has now established normal, upright posture over a controlled hip. Beginning with bridging, exercises have been working steadily towards this end and at no time has the patient's affected arm been left out of the development patterns. Normal upright posture over a controlled hip *must* be established before normal controlled walking can be expected. Remember that the elderly, frail or otherwise disabled person may achieve the desired result of balancing over alternate knees with the help of two stools (Fig. 73).

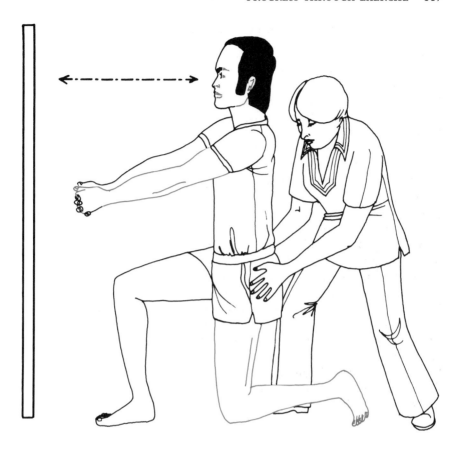

Fig. 77 Learning to balance on alternate knees

Figure 78*: Propping on hands with shoulders rolled outwards

With some patients this exercise may be taught and used much earlier in the rehabilitation programme. It is a useful way of getting the patient to stand on his hand. As shown in the illustration, he is standing firmly on the required, correctly positioned base. The exercise should be introduced as soon as you find the patient can do it — even if, at first, he is only successful because you are supporting his affected elbow and hand in the correct position.

As soon as the patient has been thoroughly stabilised in this position it makes a useful starting position for exercise. For example, if a solitaire board is placed on his affected side, he will stand firmly on the affected hand *without altering its position*, lean on it, lift his sound hand and rotate his body across to the affected side to reach the solitaire board. He may be taught to return to the starting position between each move he makes on the board. The lower trunk rotation involved also helps to reduce any tendency to leg spasticity.

Even after good balance has been achieved, the starting position as illustrated ought to continue to be used, as are all other balance positions marked with a star (*), to give *gentle* stabilising exercise as described under Figure 66.

Where *rolling to propping on the elbow* (Fig. 48) and *propping on hands with shoulders rolled outwards* (Fig. 78) are well-established and used in every exercise session, the patient is well set on the road to recovery.

Figure 79: Propping and rocking forwards over hands

This is a more advanced exercise and certainly the patient will not be ready to attempt it earlier than illustrated in this exercise programme. If he is to progress to controlled hand movements, the patient must continue with the rocking movement over his hands that he began in crawling exercise. Again, this is quite simply following the development of controlled movement seen in the infant. The infant gets rid of the primitive flexion grip of his fingers that he is born with in this way. Remember, this is why your patient must not be given a ball to squeeze in the early days after his stroke. Squeezing a ball simply uses the early (and now unwanted) primitive *reflex* grip and will not lead to controlled movement and the ability to straighten his fingers will be lost for ever.

From Figure 68 onward, the daily session of exercise in crawling will have continued and the performance should have improved. By now the patient should be transferring his weight well from side to side and taking good even steps forwards. He may also be ready to begin crawling backwards. Arm support is continued as long as it is necessary. When it is no longer necessary the patient is ready to begin the exercise as illustrated in Figure 79: rocking forwards and *backwards* over his hands.

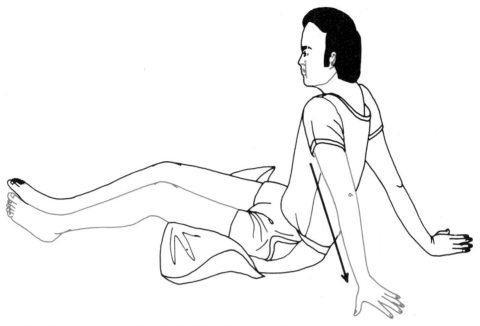

Fig. 78 Propping on hands with shoulders rolled outwards

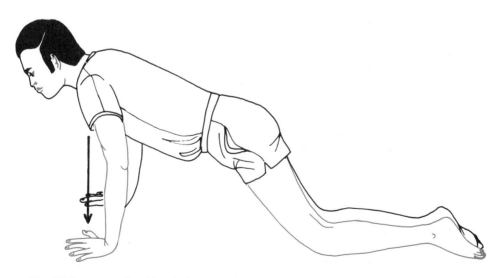

Fig. 79 Propping and rocking forwards over hands

Figure 80 (a and b): Getting up from floor on to stool

Note. Remember in the early days the help of two people may be necessary to assist the patient to get up from the floor. In this case, he will get up from lying on his back. The helpers place themselves on each side of him and, each taking a firm handshake grasp of his hands and using their other hands under his arms, they assist him into the sitting position (knees bent up as for bridging) and raise him up into the full standing position. The affected arm and shoulder will not hurt if correct procedures have been followed from the beginning and if, while raising him upwards, his shoulder is properly positioned forward and rolled into external (or outward) rotation. As rehabilitation continues, and as a progression, he may be taught to roll from his back over to elbow propping and to get up on to his knees. From this position, again helped by two people, it is a relatively easy exercise for him to get up on to his feet provided the rehabilitation programme has followed the stages suggested here.

Again, if the treatment programme has so far followed and achieved all the exercise positions suggested here, at this stage getting up from the floor does not present any problem. The patient has learnt to balance in the stand kneeling position and the solid piece of furniture (e.g. as illustrated, wooden stool or low coffee table) suggested for use when getting him down on to the floor will again be used. From the stand kneeling position alongside the stool, he places his sound hand firmly on the stool, lifts his sound leg forwards to place the foot firmly on the floor, and, leaning forwards, he pushes on the sound hand and foot, raises his buttocks and pivots round into a sitting position. The diagrams are self- explanatory.

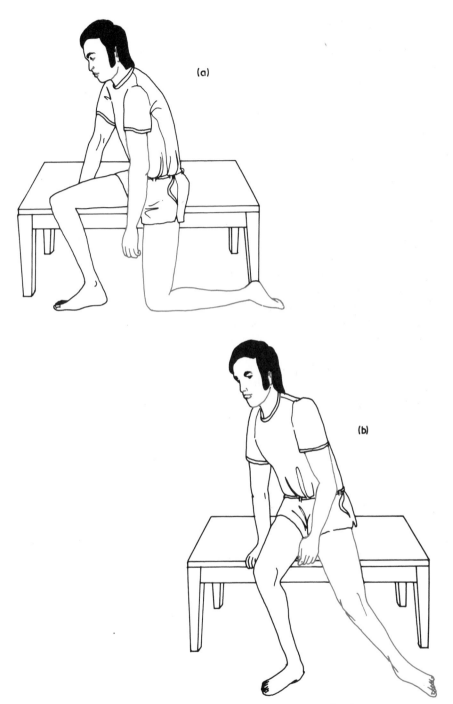

Fig. 80 (a & b) Getting up from floor on to stool. The helper may find it necessary to hold the patient's affected hand (using the handshake grasp)

Figure 81*: Stabilising in sitting

Sitting balance ought to have been established early in the treatment programme (see Figs 28 and 35). However, a continuing daily session in balance training in the sitting position ought to be given all through rehabilitation. This is because it helps to *use* and *gain control* of all the postural reflexes — or the reflexes which lead to controlled posture.

Figure 81 gives another self-explanatory diagram and the suggested exercises ought to be faithfully carried out, not only as a means of stimulating postural reflexes, but, as a very suitable way of approaching weight-bearing over a correctly positioned hand. This is probably an appropriate place to list the points that must be remembered in all stabilising exercises:

1. Use a mirror wherever possible. The patient ought to be able to see his head and shoulders, if not his whole body.

2. The affected arm and leg must not be allowed to drift or move out of the recovery pattern into the spasticity pattern.

3. Any pressure given by the helper must be gentle, must build up slowly and must be withdrawn slowly. It must not be allowed to send either of the affected limbs into spasticity.

4. Wherever necessary support must be given by the helper to the affected limbs — usually, at this stage, the arm.

5. Otherwise, any hand contact made by the helper's hand on the patient's body will be made to gain the response of a returning pressure from the patient and will therefore be on the side to which he is expected to push, or lean. In other words, if he is expected to push, or lean, towards his affected side the helper's hand will be placed on (and will push gently from) his affected side. *Do not place your hand on his sound side and pull him across to his affected side.* This would simply produce a stronger lean towards his sound side.

6. If in any doubt about the *right* way to assist the patient in stabilising exercises, ask for the advice of the physiotherapist.

Note. A very useful treatment aid is found in a stool (approximately of the size illustrated) that is built with lateral rockers (or one adapted by a clever joiner). Sitting, as positioned in Figure 81, the patient learns to rock from side to side. He may also turn towards his affected side, place his sound hand parallel with his affected hand, and rock gently over both hands. The value of such an exercise has already been explained.

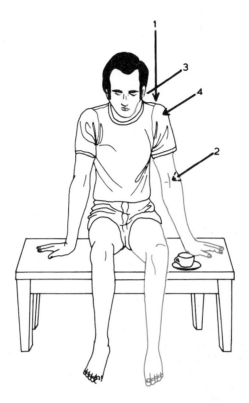

Fig. 81 Stabilising in sitting, the helper uses both of her hands to give:
(a) *1 & 2* Gentle pressure downwards from shoulder to hand with elbow support.
(b) *3* Gentle pressure to the back of the head to give spinal extension, or thrust, in the arms.
(c) *4* Gentle pressure laterally at the shoulder will finally maintain position.

Figure 82: A useful resting position

This is a useful resting position because, even if the patient is apparently 'resting', he is sitting in a good position. (He is living in the correct pattern.) His head, shoulders, hips and knees are all well within the recovery pattern. As he sits and 'rests' he is weight-bearing forwards over his feet and elbows, both being used as the correctly positioned base already described. Thus, he is weight-bearing correctly through his hip and thigh and through his shoulder, and both hip and shoulder joints are correctly maintained in a very acceptable position. He may also use this 'resting' position as a starting position for exercise, e.g. an object may be placed on the table, out of his reach unless he stretches forwards to touch it with his knuckles. He may be asked to stretch forwards and push the object across the table and, as he withdraws from his point of furthest stretch, his helper returns the object to its original position. If his starting position is correct and his feet are placed so that his knees are bent to 90°, as he reaches forwards he transfers his weight well forward over his heels. To prevent boredom his helper may count the number of times he pushes the object, challenging him to beat his record of the previous treatment. This ought not to be done to the point of frustration. A clever helper will think up alternative 'games'.

Figure 83: Sitting at table as in previous figure

1. Trunk rotation

Sitting, as shown in the previous figure, the patient may also practise upper trunk rotation. He keeps his hands clasped, thumbs uppermost, elbows straight and sweeps his hands in an arc from side to side (Arrow 1).

2. Arm rotation

Remembering that the affected arm is mobilised into external rotation (recovery pattern) he is also very well-placed at the high table to practise arm rotation. This means that he uses the sound hand to assist the affected hand into the correct rotation movement (Arrow 2). When the arm is in full external, or outward, rotation the hand faces upwards to the ceiling.

Note As already stated (notes given for Fig. 17) it is an essential part of good rehabilitation to give the patient self-care exercises. This is part of handing over the care of his own limbs to him and this should be done wherever possible. Figures 82–83 show how (sitting well-positioned for resting periods) it is possible to turn a good resting position into an exercise position where the patient may do something useful for himself. It should therefore not be left until late on in the treatment programme. It should be introduced as soon as possible and should continue to be used as arm function recovers.

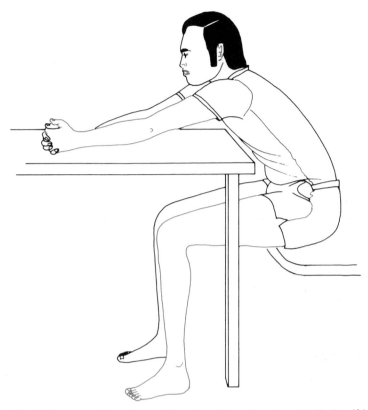

Fig. 82 A very useful resting position that will greatly assist rehabilitation if incorporated into much of the resting time (Sitting at a lower table, hands clasped and leaning on the elbows may also be used to great advantage)

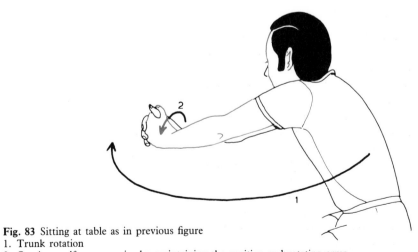

Fig. 83 Sitting at table as in previous figure
1. Trunk rotation
2. Continue self-care exercise by maintaining the position and rotating arms

Figure 84 (a and b): Standing up

This is an exercise which follows the previous one in a natural sequence. Reaching forwards to stretch across the table is readily changed to reaching forwards towards the floor if the table is removed. It is essential for the patient to get his weight well forward over his feet if he is going to stand up successfully by himself. He has already transferred his weight forward over his heels while sitting at the table. Now he transfers it still further forward as he reaches his hands towards the floor. As he gains confidence in reaching forwards, he should be encouraged to take more and more weight through his feet until he finds he can stand on his feet and lift his buttocks a few inches off his seat. With continued practice he will learn to lift his buttocks higher and higher until he gains an upright posture.

Note. The patient *leans forward into standing.* In other words, he must transfer his centre of gravity forward over his feet if he is to stand successfully. The patient who leans backwards will never learn to stand up unaided.

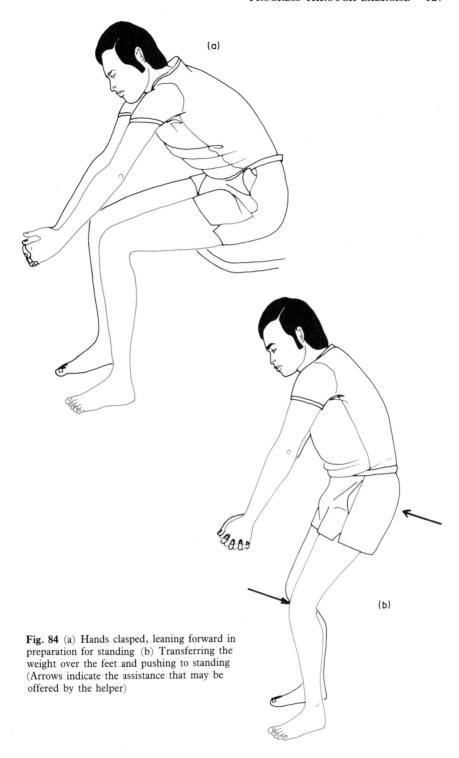

Fig. 84 (a) Hands clasped, leaning forward in preparation for standing (b) Transferring the weight over the feet and pushing to standing (Arrows indicate the assistance that may be offered by the helper)

Figure 85 (a to e): Getting into a bath

This figure gives a stage by stage description of a suggested way of getting into a bath. Even so, most patients will find it necessary to have a helper standing by ready to give assistance where necessary. But, if the method illustrated is used, the assistance that is needed will be minimal and bathing may be fairly quickly established with the minimum of fuss while the patient is allowed to feel as independent as possible. A fairly wide variety of bath aids — bath stools, boards, mats etc. — are to be had but the assistance of the expert will be necessary in the beginning and she will be able to give sound professional advice on the best aids that ought to be supplied for each individual patient. This is generally done by the occupational therapist.

The following description will be found to be suitable for most patients. Getting in and out of the bath may at first present problems. Properly handled it becomes a simple exercise and purely a repetition of a feat which has already been established. It follows the same sequence as getting in and out of bed.

A non-slip rubber mat is placed in the bottom of the bath and an adjustable bath seat is placed inside the bath. At this stage, time may be very well spent on a few trial attempts at getting in and out of a dry bath with the patient fully dressed. This allows him to concentrate on the actions he must make rather than turning his thoughts to water and the need to wash. If correct handling has been instituted from the beginning there is usually no serious problem.

A chair or stool is correctly positioned beside the bath so that the patient sits side-on to the bath with his sound hand next to the bath (Fig. 85a). If the bath is alongside a wall, so that it is not possible to approach it from either side, it is *not* necessary to consider where the taps are placed; it is essential to have the patient's sound side correctly placed. If he has to sit with his back to the taps it cannot be helped. When he reaches the stage of getting into a full bath, the water must be run before he gets in and the hot tap must not drip on his back. Modern methods of heating water may lead to a dripping tap that is unbearably hot. The taps should be padded with a towel in case the patient leans backwards.

To get into the bath the patient is taught to follow the illustrated sequence:

1. He places his sound hand on the side of the bath, stands and pivots a quarter turn to sit down on the edge of the bath (Fig. 85b).

2. He then pushes on his hand and slides his buttocks over the edge of the bath on to the bath seat (Fig. 85c). His helper may hold his affected arm in a good position and assist the transfer to the bath seat.

3. Next he transfers his sound hand to the opposite side of the bath, or ideally to a handrail on the opposite side of the bath or on the wall, and lifts the sound leg into the bath (Fig. 85d).

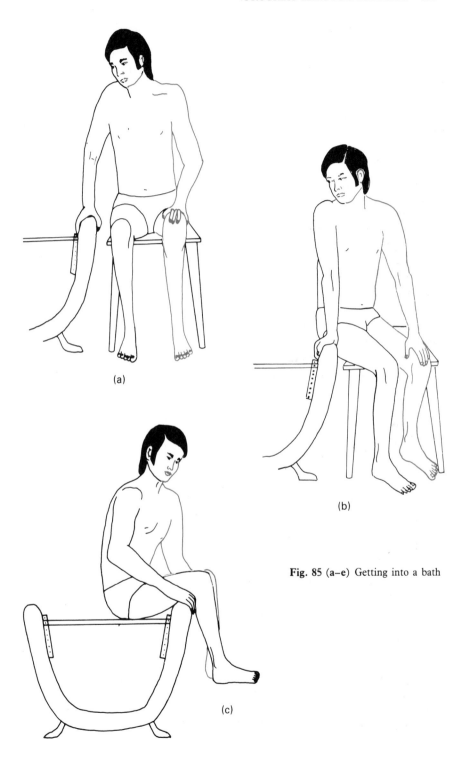

(a)

(b)

(c)

Fig. 85 (a–e) Getting into a bath

4. He removes his sound hand from the handrail and assists his affected leg into the bath (Fig. 85e).

For bathing, a suitable mixing spray for hair washing fastened to the bath taps with the water set at the right temperature will assist the patient's independence, as will a rubber soap sticker fastened to the edge of the bath so that he does not lose the soap. The aim to help him to live in the recovery pattern will be further helped if the soap is placed on his affected side. Thus, every time he reaches for the soap he will rotate, or roll, over his hips towards his affected side. To begin with, the bath seat may be used at its full height and the patient may bath on it sitting above the water. As rehabilitation makes progress the bath seat will be lowered until he reaches the time when he can readily transfer from the seat to the bottom of the bath. The seat will then be removed altogether while he is in the bath but it will be placed in position again to assist him when he is ready to get out. The procedure for getting out of the bath is a repetition in reverse: Figure 85e–a.

Note on dressing. Dressing may present problems. Where this is simply a physical difficulty of getting affected limbs into clothing, or one-handed fastening of buttons, the necessary help should be given to prevent spasticity build-up, particularly in the affected arm, and to prevent build-up of frustration. Where, on the other hand, it is a perceptual problem, the help of the expert in rehabilitation will surely be needed. To help you to understand a little about the perceptual problem study the notes given with Figure 1. Remember that your patient may not recognise his clothes (agnosia), or he may have difficulty in performance (apraxia), or in both. Familiar objects may not be recognised, so the patient may be physically capable of dressing but unable to recognise his clothes or remember how to put them on. *Frustration must not be allowed to take over or progress will go backwards instead of forwards.* In this case your patient must be given simple tasks that he is able to accomplish and no excessive demands must be made of him.

Where there is a perceptual problem, the patient may also have difficulty in feeding himself. He may not even recognise a spoon or understand its purpose. But, if rehabilitation is approached by careful nursing with good positioning at all times, by an advancing exercise programme as suggested here, and, where possible, by a cheerful and hopeful approach from the occupational therapist, these apraxic difficulties will lessen.

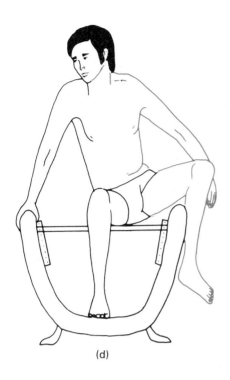

(d)

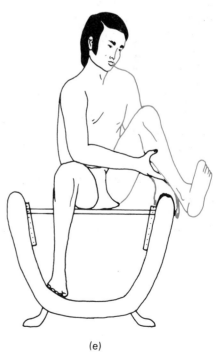

(e)

Figure 86: Controlled walking

This figure shows walking which is being controlled by the physiotherapist from the level of the patient's hips. The method illustrated is useful for a nervous patient who is in the early stages of walking re-education. It gives him something to hold on to while his affected arm is maintained in a good position. The physiotherapist is gripping his forearms with her upper arms while, at the same time, she is giving supporting control to his hips. He has to learn to step forward *over* the affected hip with a sideways and forward movement, and the physiotherapist is well-placed to assist this correct forward and lateral transference of his weight. In other words, he has to learn to transfer his weight over a correctly positioned foot (as already described) and the assistance given here by the physiotherapist will ensure that the desired movement takes place. This walking exercise may also be practised with the patient's arms placed up on the physiotherapist's shoulders, or she may walk behind him giving supporting hip control from behind while he walks with his hands clasped at the front. Again, in all three of these possible supporting positions, the hip controlled assistance emphasises the lateral forward movement over the affected hip.

If the earlier stages of stand kneeling and balancing over the affected hip and knee have been carefully taught, moving on to controlled walking should give little trouble. (See notes on Fig. 72.) Step by step, all through the beginning series of exercises, the aim has been to establish normal upright posture over a controlled hip. Beginning with bridging, exercises have been working steadily towards this end. *Normal upright posture over a controlled hip* **MUST** *be established* before normal controlled walking can be expected. Where the home helper understands the reasoning behind the exercise sequence, she will find there is much she can do to help further the rehabilitation programme. Wherever possible, the physiotherapist will hand over to her. It should also never be forgotten that, wherever possible, the patient should also be taught the reasoning behind the positions and the exercises he will be expected to learn if he is to make the best of rehabilitation.

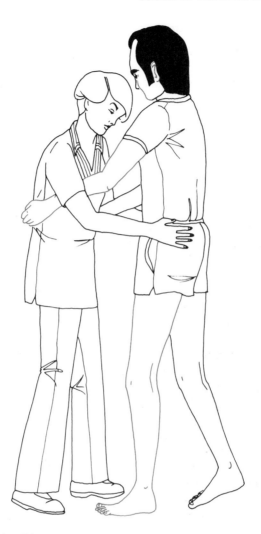

Fig. 86 Controlled walking

Figure 87: A useful hold to control walking

This hold may be used to control walking as balance progresses. This figure illustrates my own particular favourite supporting hold for walking the stroke patient. I like it because the patient's affected arm is well positioned, weight being transferred from the externally rotated shoulder down through an extended elbow to the heel of the hand. Note the handshake grasp given to the patient, keeping his thumb uppermost to maintain external rotation of the shoulder. This leaves the helper's other hand free to control his body position. She extends her wrist and extends and spreads all her fingers and her thumb to give maximum contact between the back of her hand and his lateral chest wall and his upper arm; at the same time she maintains his elbow extension with her upper arm. This puts her in an ideal position to control his body movement and assist in the correct transference of his weight over his affected hip as he steps forwards on to the affected foot. I find that where this position is properly used correct walking is quickly established and correct weight transference does not usually give any trouble. *But,* here the tall helper is at a disadvantage and she will find she cannot easily place her free hand (the right hand as illustrated here) up under her patient's arm in the required position. The tall helper would be advised to use one of the other walking holds. It is important to note that *controlled walking is never led from the patient's sound side.*

As has already been said, handling the patient from his sound side does not lead to controlled movement and, in this instance, would not lead to a normal controlled gait. The patient would lean to his sound side towards his helper and very soon he would be using his affected leg as little more than a second-rate prop. He would not transfer his weight properly through his affected leg and this would mean that he would weight-bear through the front part of his foot and not through his heel. This would quickly build-up the unwanted action of the dominant reflexes. His affected hip would turn out into external rotation (spasticity pattern) and he would never walk again with a normal gait. The spasticity pattern would take over.

Note. Figure 108e shows another useful handgrip which may be used to assist the patient to walk. This handgrip not only helps to control transference of weight over to the affected side, but also gives valuable weight-bearing through a well-positioned arm (heel of hand to shoulder). By this stage in the rehabilitation programme, the patient should be on his feet for several exercise periods a day. Choose the hall, or the most spacious place available for walking practice and walk the patient up and down many times. When turning, always teach him to turn towards his weak side. Handled as suggested here, it is a thoroughly therapeutic exercise and he will soon be ready to have a go outside. But, before he goes outdoors, he ought to be thoroughly stabilised in standing (see notes on Fig. 91).

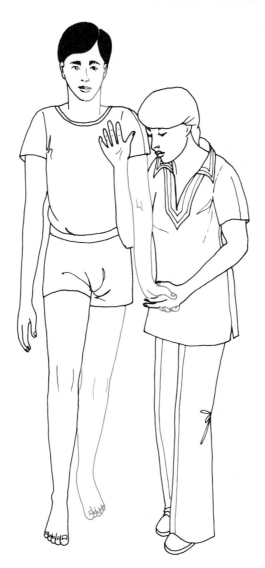

Fig. 87 A useful hold to control walking

Figure 88: Leaning on forearms, knee bending and stretching

Figure 88 shows forearm support after the position has been well stabilised. Remember, tilting the head backwards helps to stabilise the position (see Fig. 4: 2nd month) and the helper may increase the rehabilitation value of the exercise by giving pressure down through the shoulder in the direction indicated by the arrow. Once the position is thoroughly stabilised, the patient will be able to maintain the position of his affected forearm without help and his shoulders will not sag. While in this position the patient should also be taught to practise rocking backwards and forwards over his forearms and he should rock from side to side, again transferring his weight right over the affected side. Note the correct parallel position of the forearms. He should also practise knee bending and stretching. All exercises are rehabilitating arm and leg simultaneously.

Figure 89: Leaning on the hands

Progressing from leaning on the forearms, the patient should now be taught to push down on his hands and straighten his elbows. To begin with it will probably be necessary to support his affected hand firmly in position (digits spread out, particularly the thumb) and also to support his elbow. It will also be necessary to emphasise that he straightens his elbows by *pushing down on his hands*. The heel of his affected hand must remain firmly in position and elbow support should not be withdrawn until he can do the movement correctly without help. When he is able to stand (as shown in Fig. 89, with or without supporting help) he should be taught to rock backwards and forwards over his hands. He will not free the primitive flexor grip (remember the newly born infant) and release his hand for functional movement unless he does this.

While in this position he should also practise knee bending and stretching. He should do this for two reasons:

1. It will increase the value of the arm exercise by increasing the weight that is transferred through the heel of his affected hand.

2. It will strengthen the action of his affected knee and help towards knee control. (Remember that elbow and knee recovery overlap with the later hand and foot recovery.)

Note. Where hand recovery is slow, particularly where spasticity is a problem, sponge rubber pieces may be used to hold the fingers and thumb widely separated for all hand weight-bearing exercise. Note, also, that the same technique may be applied to the neglected foot; widely spread toes inhibit spasticity and may allow the forefoot to clear the ground in walking. *At all times it is the best possible therapy for hand recovery if the helper is able to support the affected hand in the full recovery pattern for all weight-bearing exercise (Fig. 43a) until the patient is able to maintain the position himself.*

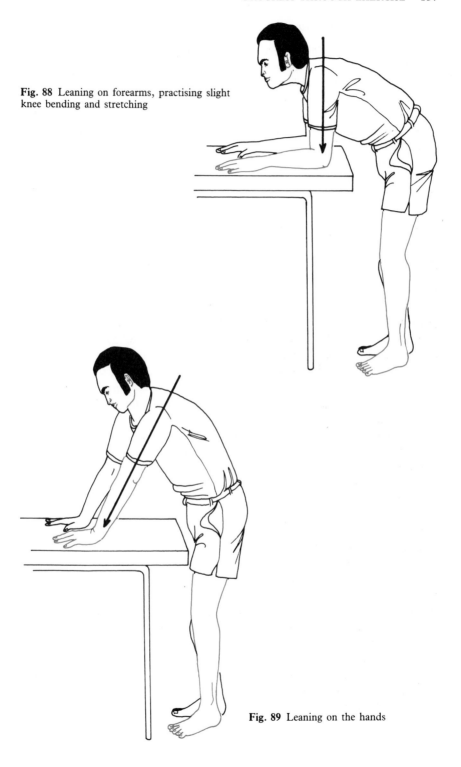

Fig. 88 Leaning on forearms, practising slight knee bending and stretching

Fig. 89 Leaning on the hands

Figure 90: Walking aids

Sooner or later it will be necessary to decide whether or not the patient ought to have the use of a walking aid. Before making this important decision, certain facts about the stroke patient and the use of walking aids ought to be understood. Then it should be possible to reach the correct decision for each individual patient.

Firstly, the method of rehabilitation presented in this book makes a *symmetrical approach to recovery*. The patient is not allowed to compensate for his disability by using the sound side of his body and neglecting to use his affected side. He builds his recovery round an approach that treats his body as a whole and works with the sound side across the midline to his affected side to initiate bilateral activity. Thus, if he is given a one-handed walking aid in his sound hand he will be asked to leave these sound principles of good rehabilitation behind. For, if he is given a one-handed walking aid in his sound hand, he will lean on it and on his sound leg while he circumducts the affected leg in the spasticity pattern to take a step forwards. At the same time, the effort required to move the affected leg will draw his affected arm upwards and inwards into the flexor spasticity pattern. In other words, he will not transfer his weight across to the affected side and he will never again establish a normal walking gait.

He will quite simply compensate for his disability with his sound side and the effort he makes to achieve a walking gait will lead to a huge build-up of excessive muscle tone in his affected side — *this build-up of tone following the dominant anti-gravity pattern of spasticity*. **He will become progressively more and more disabled.**

Secondly, if the method of rehabilitation presented in this book is to continue and a walking aid is thought to be necessary, *it must be two-handed* for the above reasons.

Types of walking aids

Figure 90a: The Rollator may be used as a useful adjunct to training for normal walking. With the Rollator held steady by the helper, the patient is taught to hold his stance with both arms in external rotation at the shoulders, elbows and wrists in extension. The correct arm position is easily obtained if the handgrips are lowered so that the patient is leaning forwards slightly while he grips them. His helper may hold his affected hand in position with the full length of his thumb stretched out *along the top of the handgrip*. He is then taught to lean on the heels of his hands (particularly the thumb) while he transfers his weight over his affected arm and leg, to mark time transferring his weight from side to side, to balance on alternate legs and to open and close his fingers. The Rollator may then make a very useful walking aid.

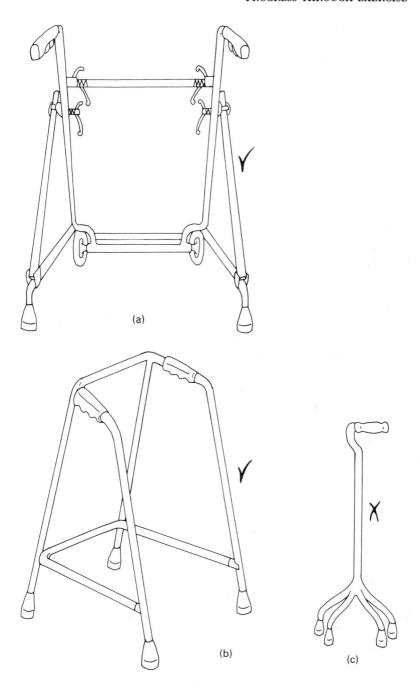

Fig. 90 Walking aids (a & b) two handed (c) one handed

Figure 90b: The Zimmer may only be used for the patient with good arm control. It must always be remembered that, unless the hand has been successfully released from the primitive flexor grip and controlled finger movements initiated, to hold a Zimmer Aid will only increase any spastic tendency.

Figure 90c: The Quadruped should not be used for the reason given above under Figure 90. The same applies to any walking stick. Such one-sided aids should only be offered where sound rehabilitation principles have been abandoned and it has to be said that such patients will inevitably be faced with increasing spasticity and ever increasing disability.

Figure 91: Standing position for stabilising

Figure 91 shows the Zimmer Walking Aid being used in good rehabilitation. Standing practising posture in front of a full-length mirror is always time well spent. Where it is not possible to have the use of a full-length mirror, the mirror used must at least give a clear image of the patient's head and shoulders. As illustrated, a way is suggested of using the smaller mirror hanging on a wall. The patient is well positioned in front of it and supported by his Zimmer Aid. As soon as he has successfully attained this position he should be stabilised in it — just as he was stabilised in all positions leading up to standing, e.g. crawling and stand kneeling. As before, he must be taught to transfer his weight laterally over the affected side and he must be taught to hold his weight evenly over *both* feet. Standing with his weight evenly distributed over both feet, his helper may then use this position to further stimulate the necessary postural reactions. He must learn to resist any pressure she gives from any direction. In other words, he maintains his starting position unmoved while she gently tries to disturb his balance. She will offer *gentle* pressure from various points (as indicated by the arrows) and her command will be: 'Don't let me move you!' Again, this must not develop into a battle of strength and at no time should she risk giving any strong pressure that will gain an undesirable response by bringing in the strong dominant reflexes of the spasticity pattern. The golden rule is to make sure the weight-bearing bases are positioned correctly and then work gently. In the early days, the helper may hold the affected thumb in position so that weight is transmitted through the correctly positioned heel of the hand.

Note. The Zimmer ought not to be used as a walking aid. This is because the patient uses a flexion pattern to grip and lift the aid forward and this will increase any tendency towards spasticity of the arm. *The standing position for stabilising* as described under Figure 91 would be more suitably undertaken with the Zimmer discarded and the hands correctly positioned with the patient leaning on a table — see weight-bearing over a correctly positioned base (Fig. 43) and this should progress to stabilising in standing with no hand support.

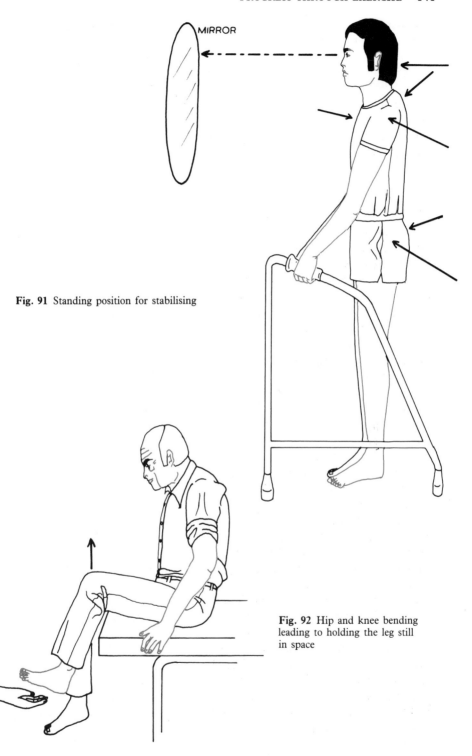

MIRROR

Fig. 91 Standing position for stabilising

Fig. 92 Hip and knee bending leading to holding the leg still in space

Figure 92: Hip and knee bending leading to holding the leg still in space

Figure 92 has been included as a reminder of the stages rehabilitation has been following. By now the patient ought to be able to do the following:

1. Recognise the position of his limb in space.
2. Move the limb in space.
3. Support and hold the limb in space.

If he cannot do any one (or all) of these three things the advice of the physiotherapist may be needed. She should be able to isolate his difficulty, perhaps step up earlier intensive training and advise on future home care. **From the earliest days, each progression on treatment should be mastered before the next is undertaken.**

Figure 93: Practising steps before climbing stairs

In the position illustrated, the patient is well-placed to practise left-sided lateral transfer of his body weight while he lifts his sound foot on and off the step. The back of an armchair is being used to support his forearms and a suitable box makes the step. This leaves the helper in a position to watch her patient's performance and to make sure he transfers his weight right over to his affected side. If he does the movement correctly he will take his weight through his affected foot and through his affected forearm as he lifts his sound foot. At first she may find it necessary to use both of her hands to support his hips so as to help him to make the necessary forward and lateral movement over his affected hip while he lifts the sound foot up on to the step. This is quite a demanding exercise for the patient when it is done properly. It needs a very positive sideways and forward movement over the affected hip and may be practised over and over again to advantage, the patient lifting his sound foot up and down while the helper supports and encourages the correct hip movement. She may then support his affected knee as illustrated by the arrows and ask him to practise mild bending and stretching of the affected knee while he keeps his sound foot on the step. She may next ask him to step right up on to the box, bringing his affected foot up beside his sound foot. A little pressure to the front of the forward knee will assist, helping the patient to stretch up over the sound foot and lift his affected foot up on to the box. As a later progression he will step up, leading with his affected foot. From this position, graduated pressure in front of, and behind, the forward knee, while he is again asked to do knee bending and stretching will provide a very useful knee strengthening exercise. Finally a little pressure to the forward knee will be used to help him to stretch up over his affected foot and bring his sound foot up on to the box beside his affected foot.

The patient who has managed to follow through rehabilitation as suggested here and has come this far, exercising and living in the recovery

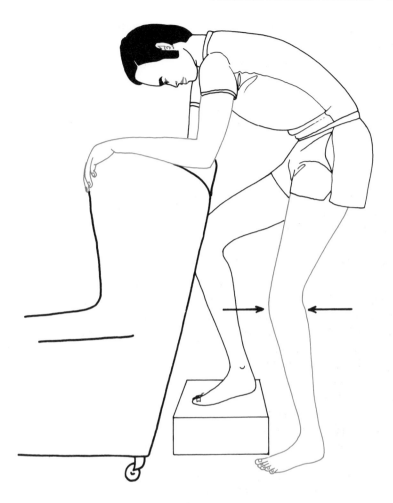

Fig. 93 Practising steps before climbing stairs

pattern and learning, step by step, to stabilise and maintain balance in each of the required positions will have come a long way along the road to recovery. But he may have failed; he may have fallen by the wayside. Perhaps the rehabilitation programme has defeated him. In this case, could anything more have been offered to him? To answer this question a further chapter on rehabilitation will be necessary.

6

Arm rehabilitation: extra help for the arm

Developing spasticity, in spite of meticulous positioning, may sometimes pose problems, particularly in the arm. Or, at the other end of the scale, the heavy, floppy limb with greatly diminished muscle tone may also represent a serious hurdle in the way of recovery of function. In either case, developing shoulder pain will put a stop to the necessary rolling to propping exercise routines that lead to a return of controlled movement. So, in either case, arm rehabilitation may be lagging and the patient may be in need of extra help if he is to work right through the rehabilitation programme successfully.

Can anything be done to give extra help?

Indeed it can. Perhaps one of the most helpful aids to recovery has been left until the end. If it has, it has been left because it can only be offered for home care where the home team understands all that is written in this book and is able to give adequate supporting assistance to the specialist in rehabilitation. The specialist must assess the situation and offer the extra help where and when it is required — and it is frequently required very early in the recovery programme. The arm must not be allowed to lag behind or very soon it will effectively put an end to all worthwhile treatment.

Does the patient's leg make a better recovery than his arm?

Unfortunately this is often so. In the majority of stroke cases the patient's arm recovery lags far behind his leg recovery *unless* specialised extra care is given to speed up recovery in the arm.

Why should this be?

Some clues that help to answer this question have already been given. They can be listed under three headings.

1. The urgent need to maintain the limbs in the inhibiting or recovery pattern twenty-four hours a day.
2. The need to weight-bear over a correctly positioned base.
3. The need to increase, or step up, the sensory messages which lead to controlled movement.

If these three points are considered in greater detail, the answer to this question becomes very clear.

1. *Maintaining the limbs in the recovery pattern*

It is very much easier to maintain the leg in the recovery pattern — or the correct anti-spasticity pattern — all through the day. The patient spends much of his time in sitting and, as soon as the leg positioning is properly understood, it becomes a simple matter to insist on maintenance of good sitting habits for the affected leg. It is more difficult to insist on the maintenance of a good arm pattern. Almost all stroke patients tend to hug or 'nurse' the affected arm by holding it cradled by the sound arm in a thoroughly bad and harmful position. Even during treatment sessions it is often found to be easier to maintain a correct leg pattern while faults may be made in the arm pattern, not enough care being taken over shoulder positioning.

2. *Weight-bearing over a correctly positioned base*

Again, it is a relatively easy exercise to stand on a correctly positioned foot with weight transmitted through the heel while it is much more difficult to undertake an adequate amount of standing on a correctly positioned forearm and hand, or on a correctly positioned hand. The patient will stand every time he gets out of bed, goes to the loo, or is assisted in correct walking — and he will weight-bear in sitting and standing correctly if he is properly handled and taught from the beginning, but he will probably only stand on his hand in short exercise sessions once or twice a day.

3. *Stepping up the sensory messages which lead to controlled movement*

Sensory messages must go in to the brain if a motor response is to come out. In other words, if sensory cues are deficient, or missing, there can be no purposeful controlled movement. Sensory messages are received through pressure on muscles and joints every time the patient stands up and, as suggested in (2) above, the patient stands on his lower limb much more than he does on his upper limb. This was not true in the early days of movement development of the infant. The patient also weight-bears heavily on the broad base of his buttocks and thighs if he is taught to sit correctly with his weight over both thighs, while any weight-bearing on the forearm tends to be minimal and light. Even in rolling, his lower limbs are subjected to more pressure on muscles than his upper limbs. Sensory nerve endings in joints and muscles respond accordingly. The eyes, with the help of a mirror, add more sensory messages which also assist recovery of an upright posture — upright with the patient standing on two legs but not standing on his hands!

It is probably not necessary to continue with this catalogue of reasons why leg recovery may far outstrip arm recovery in the stroke patient. What is necessary, and urgently necessary, is to find a way of boosting arm recovery and, to do this, it is necessary to find a treatment aid which will make up for the difficulties encountered in arm rehabilitation. This means that the affected arm must be given an equal chance with the affected leg.

How can this be done?

Let us once more consider the three points listed above and in doing this we find that each point leads to another question.

1. Maintaining the affected limbs in the recovery pattern so as to inhibit the dominant reflexes. Is there a treatment aid which would make a useful contribution to arm positioning while shoulder rehabilitation take place? Yes, there is.

2. Weight-bearing over a correctly positioned base. Is there a treatment aid which would make it easier to weight-bear through the arm during treatment sessions? Again, yes, there is.

3. Stepping up sensory messages through muscles and joints. Is there a treatment aid which would step up these sensory messages by means of pressure? And again, yes, there is a very effective and simple aid which takes care of these three points and which makes arm rehabilitation possible.

So what is the treatment aid that answers these problems?

The answer is found in the orally inflatable *pressure* splint. This orally inflatable arm splint is made of clear plastic casing forming a double sleeve. When the splint is fitted to the arm and fully inflated *orally* (just like a balloon), pneumatic cushioning conforms to the shape of the limb, holding it immobile and suspended to give full support with *all over even pressure*. If the limb is carefully positioned in the full anti-spasticity or recovery pattern, and the finger-tips are well back from the open end so that the fingers' ends are well included in the all over pressure, the pressure splint may be used as the perfect treatment aid. It supplies the missing answer to the three questions above. Properly used, it makes arm rehabilitation possible and, in some cases, arm recovery may even outstrip leg recovery. Again, to understand this, it might be helpful to return to the three questions that were asked above.

1. *Is there a treatment aid which would make a useful contribution to arm positioning while shoulder rehabilitation takes place?*

Yes, with a pressure splint in place, holding the arm immobile in the full inhibiting position and giving supporting stability, it becomes possible to work the shoulder in a series of carefully planned exercises which lead towards shoulder stability and controlled movement. Remember that trunk and *shoulder* recover before the elbow and hand and treatment must work towards this correct sequence.

2. *Is there a treatment aid which makes it easier to weight-bear through the arm during treatment sessions?*

Yes, with the supporting stability given by a pressure splint, weight-bearing from the heel of the hand to a correctly positioned shoulder is at once possible and easily carried out during treatment sessions. Remember that weight-bearing is an essential part of stroke rehabilitation.

3. *Is there a treatment aid which steps up sensory messages by means of deep pressure?*

Yes, obviously a splint which offers all over pressure to the affected limb must be considered as an effective rehabilitation tool. As exercises are carried out, the depth of pressure will fluctuate slightly making the sensory messages more effective.

Note. When properly applied, the pressure splint will help to relieve spasticity by maintaining the limb fully in the inhibiting pattern, *but* it will not aid the return of controlled movement unless it is used in a series of carefully chosen exercises which follow the lines of treatment already presented in this book. Exercise gives movement within the tissues and exercise given under pressure must be more effective. Allow resting time in the splint before starting exercises.

Application of the splint

The pressure splint is applied with the shoulder in external rotation and with the elbow, wrist and fingers stretched out straight, thumb pointing outwards. That is, the arm is held fully in the inhibiting or recovery pattern. The importance of this arm position cannot be stressed too often. If the wrist is bent backwards while the splint is in position (and it is important to note that this particular manipulation does not hurt if it is started *very early* in the rehabilitation programme) the *complete* inhibiting pattern is in use and the stiff wrist that so often hampers good rehabilitation will be avoided. Even if the arm seems to be completely floppy with no obvious signs of spasticity to be seen, the splint should be used. The earlier it is introduced in the treatment programme the better. It may be applied to advantage two or three times a day provided the arm is correctly positioned and the finger-tips are well back from the open end. At each application it may be left on for a reasonable period — up to one hour — and the patient ought to find it gives great comfort. Initially it ought to be used by the rehabilitation experts who should assess the family situation and hand over care, or proceed with shared care, wherever possible. *The splint must only be inflated by mouth.* The power of the human lungs will not lead to overinflation and the warmth of the breath will soften and mould the plastic to conform to the limb, thus giving the essential all over *even* pressure. **The splint should be as fully inflated as the human lungs can manage to give the required deep pressure.**

The following figures give an outline of the exercise routine that should be aimed at to help the pressure splint to become a dynamic treatment aid in stroke rehabilitation.

Figure 94: Application of arm splint

Figure 94 a, b and c shows the correct application of the arm splint in easy stages. It must be applied on top of a cotton sleeve.

1. Close the zip.
2. Pull the splint onto your own arm and take a handshake grasp of the patient's affected hand.
3. Rotate the shoulder outwards, extend the elbow and pull the splint onto the patient's positioned arm (a).
4. Maintain the correct hand position as in (b), making sure that the thumb is stretched out sideways as illustrated.
5. Inflate the splint *by mouth*. Note that the long inflation tube (as illustrated in Fig. 103) makes it possible to hold the tube with your teeth leaving two hands free to manage the splint.

Warm air from the lungs warms and moulds the inner sleeve to the limb giving all over *even* pressure with no danger of constriction. The splint must be firmly inflated; the human lungs cannot over inflate. The *finger-tips must be well back from the open end* and a cotton sleeve should be worn under the plastic sleeve to prevent a sweat rash. **Never** allow your patient to sit out in the sun while wearing the splint. The splint is easiest to apply with the patient lying on his back with his knees bent up.

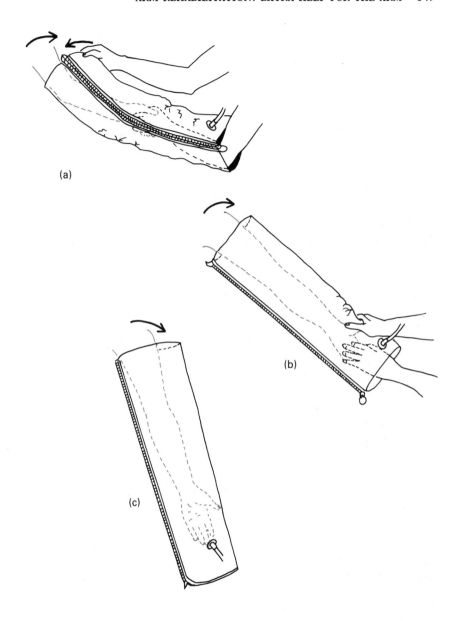

(a)

(b)

(c)

Fig. 94(a–c) Application of arm splint

Figure 95: Arm positioning

Arm positioning must include external or outward rotation of the shoulder. The thumb should point away from the patient's body and all shoulder movements should lead the thumb to point in this direction.

Figure 96: Arm elevation with pressure splint

This figure shows the desirable resting position with the splint in place. It is to the patient's advantage to rest in this position for at least twenty minutes before an exercise session begins.

Figure 97: Shoulder rehabilitation

Here, refer back to Figure 16. Now, once again, the pressure splint makes it very easy to maintain the correct arm pattern with external rotation of the shoulder while arm raising is carried out. This is one of the most important shoulder exercises. At first it is done passively — that is, the patient takes no active part and the helper moves the limb. Again, right through the movement, the patient's thumb points away from his body and it should not hurt. If it hurts, correct handling methods have not been carefully followed from the very beginning and it will help to rest in a correctly applied splint and move more gently into manipulation using a pain-free range of movement. As shown in Figure 97, this type of treatment is suitable for all age groups. The helper's hand positions have been represented here for easy illustration but note that the helper would approach the movement from the patient's affected side. The patient goes through three progressions in treatment which may take weeks to accomplish:

1. Passive Movements
2. Active Assisted Movements (he helps)
3. Active Unassisted Movements (he no longer needs help)

At the same time, these three stages lead him into holding the limb still in space without outside help other than the splint (in the position illustrated here). With the help of the full supporting pressure offered by the splint these exercise progressions are much more quickly achieved than would otherwise be possible.

Note. The bridging exercise *should be practised* while the arm splint is on and the shoulder carefully positioned in external rotation.

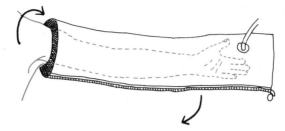

Fig. 95 Arm positioning

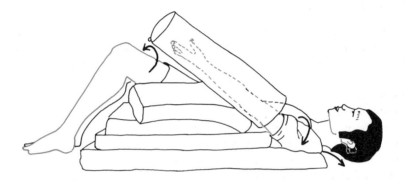

Fig. 96 Arm elevation with pressure splint

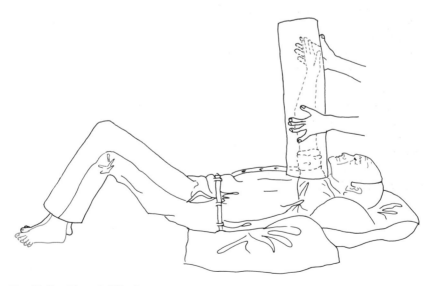

Fig. 97 Shoulder rehabilitation

Figure 98: Shoulder forward, patient pushing forwards

This figure represents another vital manipulation. The diagram is self-explanatory. The patient has been taught stabilising in side lying and he keeps his hips stationary while he moves his affected shoulder backwards and forwards. The helper may give pressure as indicated by the arrows. The patient may be positioned for resting with the splint on and the affected arm well supported on three pillows in the illustrated attitude. Note leg pattern with the hip rolled well forwards. He may also learn to 'saw' the pillows as a self-care exercise. All such early exercise will help to establish Active Unassisted Movement as in (3) on page 150.

Figure 99: Arm positioned, hip rolling with shoulder held steady

Again the patient has been stabilised in side lying and the splint supports the arm in the necessary position while he moves his lower trunk, rotating his affected hip backwards and forwards in a rolling movement. At first his helper assists the movement, then he is taught to do it by himself, and finally she resists the movement while he does a strong hip exercise rotating against her pressure. In the latter case (where strong leg exercise is practised) the arm splint is performing a very necessary function. It prevents hard exercise in any part of the body overflowing into the affected arm where it would follow the strong anti-gravity tonal pattern if the arm was not held firmly in the full inhibiting pattern. This would increase the already excessive and unwanted pattern of spasticity. In other words, the splint, by maintaining the inhibiting pattern, diverts this overflow of tone into the low tonal pattern and so assists sound rehabilitation principles and the need to restore balanced tone. The physiotherapist calls this practice 'controlling associated reactions'.

Note. As early as possible in the rehabilitation programme the patient will be helped into the full crawling position with the arm supported by the splint.

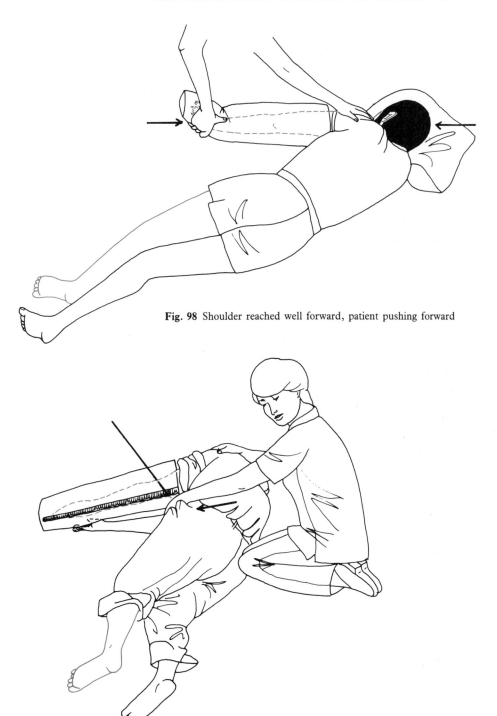

Fig. 98 Shoulder reached well forward, patient pushing forward

Fig. 99 Arm positioned, hip rolling with shoulder held steady

Figure 100: Upper trunk rotation

Here the helper is inhibiting the wrist by holding the hand position and giving resistance through the hand as the patient thrusts the hand forwards against this resistance as indicated by the arrows. He has been thoroughly stabilised in side lying and his hips do not move. The movement is a thrust from the trunk, shoulder and extended elbow to a correctly positioned hand. As illustrated, the shirt sleeve has been rolled up; remember that in practice you would leave the shirt sleeve down.

Figure 101: Shoulder care

The aim of all these exercises is first to produce *shoulder stability and controlled shoulder movement*. Failure to achieve this aim leads to failure in arm rehabilitation with no possibility of regaining a controlled and working arm. From the earliest day of rolling this aim has been in mind. Until the patient can raise his own arm to the position shown in Figure 97, and maintain it steadily in this position, he has not got shoulder stability. As soon as he has got shoulder stability he is ready to use a below the elbow (or half arm) pressure splint. But, because shoulder and elbow rehabilitation overlap, the shorter splint may be used as shown here at a slightly earlier date. Here, in Figure 101, the elbow is being held in the bent position by the helper and shoulder elevation (or reaching above the head) is being practised. This may be followed by an exercise in which the helper continues to support the position shown and helps her patient to bend and stretch his elbow.

Figure 102: Elbow rehabilitation

When shoulder stability has been established it is often a quite simple task to establish elbow stability *because*, as stated above, the progress of recovery is from shoulder to elbow to hand and this returning function overlaps. Thus, full shoulder stability establishes partial elbow stability. With the half arm splint in position, Figure 102 shows a useful way of helping to establish elbow function. The patient is taught to watch his hand while his helper does a passive exercise, performing the movement of bending and stretching his elbow by taking the palm of his hand down towards his face and back to the starting position. He will be taught to make the usual progressions from passive, too assisted active, to active movement as the elbow function improves. Again, the splint keeps the hand in the recovery pattern and away from the spasticity pattern. Note that any early active exercise the recovering elbow is able to make may, because of effort, lead to unwanted exercise overflow into the spasticity pattern of the hand. The splint is used to control this.

At this stage, when the splint is removed, a hand propping exercise ought to be given, e.g. as in Figure 78.

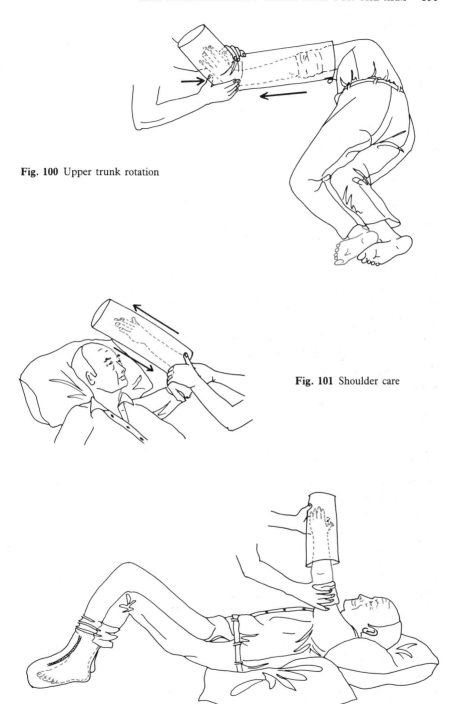

Fig. 100 Upper trunk rotation

Fig. 101 Shoulder care

Fig. 102 Elbow rehabilitation

Figure 103: Recent development in stroke splints (1986 update)

I have now used pressure splints for the last seventeen years and they have proved their worth in the clinical field many times and in many difficult rehabilitation situations. Svend Andersen plastic Industri of Denmark (and in particular Claus Jeppesen) have co- operated with me in my development of the URIAS splint stroke programme. I had tested all splints that became available over the years and settled for URIAS because they are made of a most suitable and specially developed PVC–sheeting — the inner layer, a unique soft PVC–sheet gives all–over even pressure while the outer layer gives lasting durability.

Figure 103 gives a fair idea of the progress we have made:

a. *The full arm splint*, a single chamber splint, available in 2 sizes (for the average arm and for the longer arm) used to maintain inhibiting position of elbow, wrist and fingers and to assist early weight–bearing.

b. *The half arm splint*, a single chamber splint, for use below the elbow, to maintain inhibiting position of wrist and fingers.

c. *The leg gaiter*, a double chamber splint, to support the leg in standing with inward rotation and a semi-flexed knee. See footnote. (2 sizes)

d. *The elbow splint*, a single chamber splint, to give support and stability to a weak elbow for exercise routines.

e. *The hand splint*, a double chamber splint, used to maintain the inhibiting position of the thumb and fingers for exercise routines, e.g. as in early crawling.

f. *The foot splint*, a single chamber splint which will maintain an inhibiting foot position *if it is correctly applied*.

Footnote. All the splints must have carefully correct application. The application will be described in the text as each splint is brought into the programme. The series of splints make it possible to control the patient's muscle tone in all situations while the rehabilitation programme is undertaken along the lines suggested in the section on Progress through exercise (p. 79).

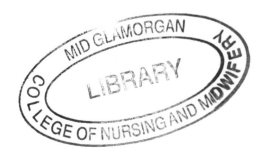

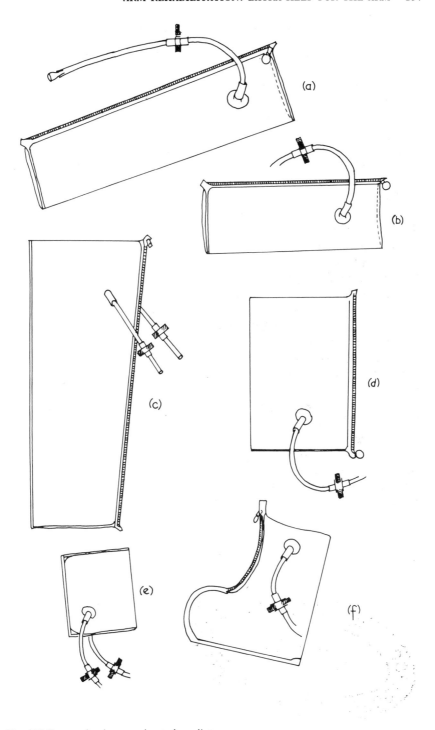

Fig. 103 Recent development in stroke splints

Figure 104: Full crawling position

Application of the full arm splint has been described (see Fig. 94). Figure 104 serves as a reminder that the stroke patient's progress through exercise is based on an attempt to follow infant development patterns. The full kneeling position should be established as soon as possible in the programme and, again, this can be achieved when the infant's sequence of development is followed. Thus, when the patient has learnt the early exercises and has learnt to roll, when he has stabilised in the starting position for bridging with the full arm splint in position and his knees firmly bent, he may be taught to *hold this knee position* while he rolls over towards his sound shoulder and continues the roll so that he finishes the movement on his knees in high kneeling (stand kneeling as in Fig. 76). (The helpher will support the affected arm and *maintain the external rotation of the shoulder* while the patient follows through the roll over onto his knees.) The helper then assists the correct placing of the affected hand as the patient lowers himself down onto both hands. Having achieved this full crawling position the patient follows the exercise programme as suggested earlier in the text (see notes on Fig. 75). Later in the programme when he is ready to crawl the full arm splint has been replaced by the hand splint to control the fingers.

Note. At all times the vulnerable shoulder must be protected and maintained in external or outward rotation if it is to remain pain free. If early care of the shoulder has been diligently observed and each rehabilitation progression carefully followed the patient ought not to have shoulder problems at this stage in his training.

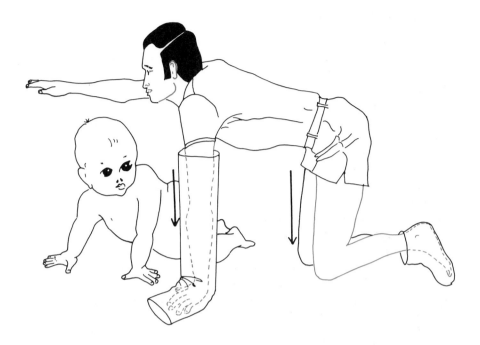

Fig. 104 Full crawling position

Figure 105: Rocking backwards and forwards

Rocking backwards and forwards on the hands is a very useful exercise. As the illustration shows, the patient is wearing three splints for elbow, hand and foot.

1. *The elbow splint*, a single chamber splint, is used to give support and stability to a weak elbow for exercise routines. It is a broad (almost square) splint designed to distribute all over even pressure which will not be harmful to circulation and is used for short exercise sessions. It is inflated by mouth (as must be all URIAS splints; the human lungs will not over-inflate) and should be placed on the arm with the zip down the inner aspect of the elbow. Inflate it by holding the zip close to the arm so that the main balloon after inflation is over the point of the elbow to give the desired elbow support.

2. *The hand splint*, a double chamber splint, is used to maintain the inhibiting position of the thumb and fingers. When placed in position on the hand with straight fingers and the thumb spread wide, the posterior section (Section 1 as illustrated) is inflated first to give firm pressure over the back of the hand to gain an extensor response in the fingers. Section 2 (as illustrated) is then given minimal inflation to give finger comfort and a thin weight-bearing pad over the palm of the hand.

3. *The foot splint*, a single chamber splint, will inhibit the foot *only if* it is correctly applied, i.e. it must be applied with the patient's heel right back in the heel of the splint as illustrated. *If it cannot be applied correctly it ought not to be used*. In that case the foot should be positioned with the help of a supporting pillow.

Figure 106: Modification of the crawling position

A modification of the crawling position may be necessary. As already suggested under Figure 70 and 71, treatment for the elderly frequently calls for modification. A way round any presenting difficulties ought to be found. Often the helper and the patient will work out possible modifications but inhibiting patterns must be maintained and pressure splints make this plan easier to execute.

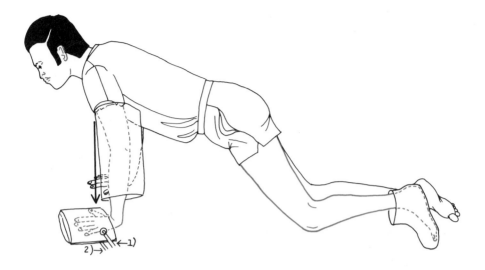

Fig. 105 Rocking backwards and forwards

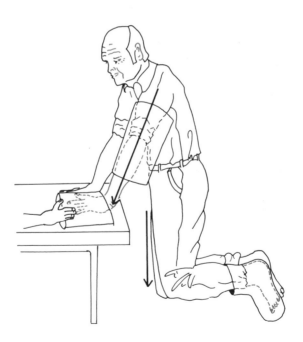

Fig. 106 Modification of the crawling position

Figure 107: Use of a leg gaiter

The leg gaiter, a double chamber splint, is used to give support and stability to the leg in standing with mild inward rotation of the leg and a semi-flexed knee. This splint is applied with the patient in standing. It is wrapped round the leg and the zip is closed having been placed so that it runs down the centre of the outer aspect of the leg as illustrated. It must be pulled as far up the leg as possible before it is inflated so that it will give firm support under the buttocks. Also, before it is inflated, the patient's foot must be positioned with the toes pointing straight forward (see Fig. 43b). *The posterior section of the splint must be inflated first* and must be fully inflated. As it is inflated the patient is encouraged to transfer his weight over to his affected side and the inflation then gently forces the knee into mild flexion and pushes the heel down into the good weight- bearing position. Finally minimal inflation is given to the anterior section of the splint giving sufficient pressure to support and give comfort over the knee. Suitably positioned, the patient then practises stepping movements *with his sound leg* while he maintains his weight over the splinted leg. Note that this is **not** a walking splint but, used as suggested here with the affected leg in this good weight- bearing position, it makes a very useful exercise splint.

Remember that the main anti-gravity tone in the lower half of the body gives a strong extensor thrust between trunk and hip with outward rotation of the hip (see Fig. 6). Weight-bearing through a limb increases muscle tone, but weight-bearing practised as suggested above with the aid of the leg gaiter applied so as to inhibit this strong anti-gravity thrust, will give a rapid advance in the rehabilitation of a good walking gait.

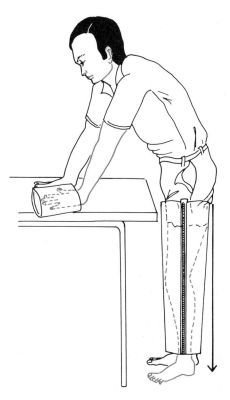

Fig. 107 Use of the leg gaiter

Figure 108: Handgrips used to work into the recovery pattern

By now it should be fully understood exactly what is meant when talking about 'working into the recovery pattern'. Where this term refers to the arm, it means that the arm works towards outward rotation of the shoulder with a straight elbow and wrist and widely separated fingers (see Fig. 8). Modifications of this recovery pattern are used, e.g. the elbow may be bent, but *at all times* some degree of outward rotation of the shoulder is maintained and measures are taken to make sure that the shoulder joint is not allowed to roll into internal rotation. Frequently, too, during exercise sessions, the wrist must be overcorrected into full extension as in crawling and weight-bearing on the palm of the hand. Understanding of this arm pattern is essential if treatment through exercise is to be properly carried out. The measures that are taken to maintain the correct shoulder pattern should use every means possible to prevent the affected hand from crossing over to the sound side of the body (and thereby allowing the affected shoulder to roll inwards). These measures have been shown to include:

1. The patient is taught to clasp his hands (thereby separating his own fingers), to bring his palms firmly together (thus rolling the shoulder still further outwards) and to keep both hands across on the affected side of his body. He is also taught, while in this position, to straighten both elbows (which rolls the shoulder still further into outward rotation).

2. When the patient sits at a table of suitable height to allow him to lean on his forearms, his forearms *must remain parallel* (to prevent the affected shoulder from turning into internal rotation). A coloured stripe may be stuck down the centre of the table to remind him that he must not allow his affected hand to stray across the line to the sound side of his body. Figure 108 is now presented to show the handgrips the helper may offer to her patient to *help him to work into the recovery pattern.*

Figure 108a: handshake. This grip is used frequently, particularly in the early days of handling the stroke patient. When the patient is lying, sitting or standing it is used in order to hold the thumb uppermost and to turn the arm away from the spasticity pattern, rotating the shoulder outwards.

Figure 108b: handshake with wrist support. Here the helper's index and middle fingers are used to give extra wrist support, preventing the wrist from bending into the spasticity pattern.

Figure 108c: recovery pattern. This grip holds the fingers and thumb in the full recovery pattern and is often used to help prevent development of the stiffy bent fingers of the spasticity pattern.

Figure 108d: weight-bearing through the heel of the hand. This grip uses the full recovery pattern of the whole hand, including full wrist extension, and turns the shoulder into full outward rotation. A very useful position in which the helper may give downward pressure from the heel of the hand to the elbow to simulate weight-bearing. It is also used to assist active elbow bending (see notes on Fig. 61). Remember that exercises should not cause pain.

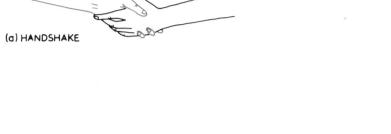

(a) HANDSHAKE

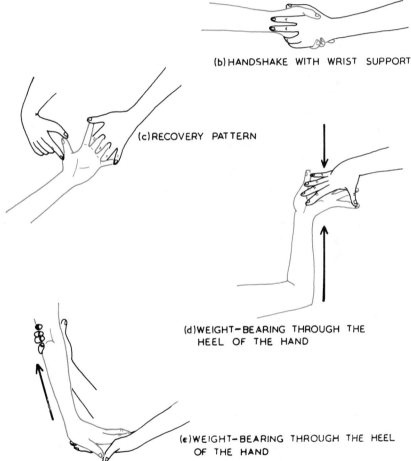

(b) HANDSHAKE WITH WRIST SUPPORT

(c) RECOVERY PATTERN

(d) WEIGHT–BEARING THROUGH THE HEEL OF THE HAND

(e) WEIGHT–BEARING THROUGH THE HEEL OF THE HAND

Fig. 108 (a–e) Handgrips used to work into the recover pattern

Figure 108e: weight-bearing through the heel of the hand. This is in many ways the most important grip of all — but all are important. This handgrip ought to be used from the very early days (see Figs 36 and 39). Obviously if it is to become an effective weight-bearing grip, the patient must be taught to transfer his weight right over to the affected side of his body. He must do this in any case if he is to achieve leg recovery and a good walking pattern, but this illustrated handgrip with added elbow support will bring about quicker rehabilitation in this essential lateral transference of body weight to the affected side. As soon as lateral transference of body weight is fully mastered, this illustrated handgrip (or a modification as in Fig. 87) ought to be used on any and every possible occasion. It means that the patient walks, weight-bearing on his affected hand as well as on his affected foot. Arm recovery usually speeds up accordingly.

Final stages in arm rehabilitation

The final stages in arm rehabilitation can only be undertaken when fully controlled shoulder and elbow movements have been re-established. This means that the patient is able to place his arm in space and hold it quite steady. In other words adequate normal muscle tone has been restored, weak muscles have been strengthened and the dominant reflexes are under control. But elbow recovery overlaps with wrist and hand recovery and so re-education of hand control has already begun. But, the final stages of rehabilitating controlled movement of the hand can only be started after the hand has been released from the primitive flexor grip. (Remember the infant's development of controlled movement and the primitive finger grip that is present at his birth). Where rehabilitation has not been carried out sufficiently to free the primitive flexor grip and release the hand for functional movement, the patient will be able to grasp an article but he will not be able to release it. In this case, the exercise programme must go right back to weight-bearing over the hand in the crawling position and continue from there.

Until this final stage in arm rehabilitation is reached, it will have been noticed that the patient has *at no time been asked to lead any activity with his affected hand* and rehabilitation has led towards the hand by means of strongly stabilising the shoulder, strongly stabilising the elbow, giving passive movements to the hand and wrist and finally re-educating movements of the elbow and hand **only when the elbow is well supported**. This takes into account the fact that recovery starts in the trunk and shoulder and moves down the arm. In this final stage, after full release of the primitive grip, the patient is ready to begin the opposite sequence where he develops controlled hand movements, and controlled hand movements lead from the hand up to the shoulder. In other words, he is at last allowed to *do things with his hand* with no fear of building up the dominant reflexes (or the spasticity pattern) which would immediately turn the shoulder into

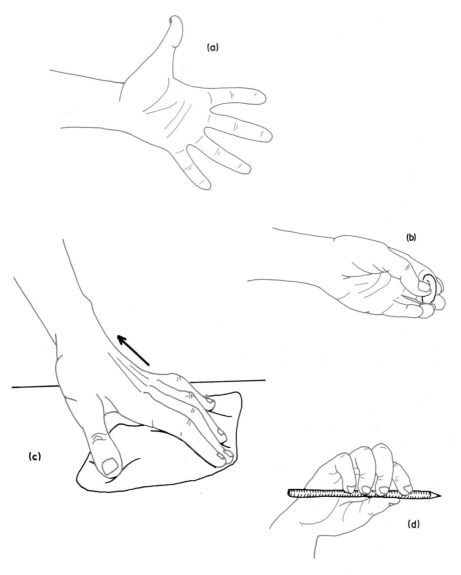

Fig. 109
(a) Fingers spread or full recovery pattern
(b) Bending to touch finger- tips
(c) Weight-bearing on finger-tips (pulling backwards against therapeutic putty)
(d) Precision movement

internal rotation and the elbow into reflex flexion. The spasticity pattern will not recur. He has restored muscle tone and his brain is in control. Figure 109 shows some of the hand movements he will be expected to perform:

a. shows his hand fully spread in the recovery pattern and held still in space.
b. shows finger bending with fine finger-tip control used to handle a small object.
c. shows straight finger control as the hand is dragged backwards through therapeutic putty.
d. shows the extreme degree of control necessary to handle a small instrument.

These diagrams are included to give an indication of the degree of recovery that is expected for a patient who is able successfully to carry through all the rehabilitation stages as represented in this book. If less than the best *must be* the end result, at least the patient will have reached the best result of which he is capable.

Suggestions to help final stages in hand rehabilitation

Sit the patient at a high table as shown in Figure 82.
    Use the exercises as given under Figures 82 and 83.
    Add on:

1. Making fists.
2. Rotating the arms (without clasped hands) so that the palms face to the ceiling
3. Rotating the affected arm as in exercise 2. Learn to do a slow, controlled movement turning the hand over and back
4. Wrists bending and stretching with hands clasped
5. Wrists bending and stretching — practised separately with hands unclasped
6. Hands pressed together in an attitude of prayer but with the fingers spread wide, wrists bending and stretching
7. Hands pressed together as in 6, keep fingers in contact and separate the palms
8. Leaning forwards with both hands turned palm downwards on the table and the fingers spread wide. Make small pulling and pushing movements
9. Place the palms over a suitable size of tin, maintain finger-tip grip on the tins and slide the tins in all directions
10. Practising precision movements of the fingers which will include pinching small pieces off a large lump of modelling putty.

The height of the table may then be changed so that the patient sits as illustrated in Figure 30. The patient sitting at the cantilever table is better placed to handle objects while his elbows are well supported. At first he weight-bears on his forearms and, as a later progression, he is taught to weight-bear on his elbows and hold his hands in the air. Using both of these positions he may practise exercises 1–7 and exercise 10 as given above. For exercise 10 he will hold the putty in his sound hand and pinch off small pieces with his affected hand. This leads into a list of exercises to be done using modelling material*:

1. The hands are pressed together in an attitude of prayer with a lump of modelling material held firmly between the heels of the hands and the palms. The patient is asked to keep the tips of his fingers together while he squeezes and moulds the modelling clay into a flattened shape. He may shift his palms slightly from side to side against each other but he must not lose finger contact. (The word 'clay' is used to cover a variety of suitable materials.)

2. Roll out a lump of clay, pressing down on the palm and keeping the fingers straight when pushing away and when pulling back.

3. Flatten a lump of clay and place the hand firmly on to it. Lift the front part of the hand off the clay but leave the heel of the hand in contact.

4. Use both hands to 'wring out' a large sausage of clay. (First make your sausage.)

5. Grip a ball of clay the size of a large orange and squeeze it to give a deep imprint, then release it, opening the hand to stretch the fingers fully out.

6. Make a clay doughnut large enough to enclose the fingers and thumb in the position shown in Figure 109b. Push open the doughnut by stretching out the fingers and thumb.

7. Place the hand flat down on a large piece of clay as shown in Figure 109c. Press the fingers down firmly into place and then pull them backward through the clay.

8. Pinch and pull out small pieces of clay from a lump held in the sound hand, using thumb and index finger, thumb and second finger, and so on.

9. Make pinch marks along the top of a strip of clay that has been rolled to a suitable thickness and pressed firmly on to the table.

10. Position the hand over a piece of clay as shown in exercise 7 but make finger-tip contact only. Again draw the hand backwards keeping firm contact.

11. Roll a very small piece of clay between the thumb and finger-tips.

As this final chapter is concerned with any extra help that may be given to push arm recovery forward, it might be useful to suggest that a suitable modelling material may be introduced into the treatment programme at an early date in the following ways:

* Various modelling materials are available for child education and play purposes and the occupational therapist uses special types of therapeutic putty. If in doubt about a suitable material to use for these exercises, advice may usually be had from the occupational therapist.

1. *In the early stages of rehabilitation.* Many patients learn quite quickly to keep their hands clasped but constantly forget to keep their *palms touching.* If your patient forgets this fine (but most important) point, he may be given a piece of thoroughly softened and moulded 'clay' to squash between his palms and the heels of his hands. He sees the lump of clay and (if sensation is intact, he also feels it) and it acts as a visual (and sensory) reminder to keep his palms and the heels of his hands firmly in contact. Every time he forgets to do this he drops the clay. This leads to quicker training and helps to establish a good handclasp position as he learns to hold on to the clay. Remember, if the palms are not in contact for many of the exercises and much of the vital positioning, the shoulder frequently rolls into the wrong rotation — inwards instead of outwards.

Plasticine is perhaps the most useful material to use at this stage.

2. *In the intermediary stages of rehabilitation.* Weight-bearing through a correctly positioned base plays a very important part at this stage of the treatment programme. A suitable clay may be used to help to establish weight-bearing through a correctly positioned hand. When the crawling position is taught and propping over the affected hand begins, the affected elbow may be supported by the helper while the affected hand is placed firmly on a flattened piece of clay. If positioning is correct, after leaning over the correctly positioned limb on to the hand, the imprint left in the clay should show firm weight-bearing through *the heel of the hand.* Where this happens it also shows that the patient's weight is being properly transferred across to the affected side of his body.

3. *In the final stages of rehabilitation.* Precision movements of the hand must be established in the final stages of rehabilitation. It would be a pity to spend a long time establishing good firm stability and control of the shoulder and elbow joints and fail to establish a good working hand. Rehabilitation frequently terminates (and is considered to be finished!) when the patient has released his hand for functional movement — in other words, when he can at last stretch out his fingers, but his hand is still weak and clumsy. It does not yet quite belong to him. The hand lacks strength, learned skills may have been forgotten and movement patterns need some re-education. This is the stage where therapeutic putty can play a leading role and the exercises suggested above may be vital to this re-education of a fully controlled hand.

It must be clear by now that any stroke rehabilitation plan will greatly benefit if pressure splints are introduced very early in the programme for the following reasons:

1. They give stability to the limb.
2. They maintain the necessary corrective positions which are used to inhibit a build up of excessive anti-gravity muscle tone.
3. They make early weight-bearing (or standing) possible — on the hands as well as the feet.

4. They divert the increase of tone produced by exercise and weight-bearing into the low tonal pattern, assisting the aim to restore balanced tone.
5. They alter and increase pressure on the limbs, giving a very positive sensory input.
6. They hastern the recovery process.

All six points lead to a possible and worthwhile recovery where each patient is given a fair chance of reaching his maximal recovery potential and a consequent reasonable quality of life.

Note that in the clinical field observation has shown that recovery may continue over a period of at least 2 years.

There are certain rules that apply to the use of pressure splints and must be observed:

1. The splints should be applied with meticulous care in every detail of corrective positioning.
2. Fingers must be fully enclosed, well back from the open end of the splint.
3. The posterior section of the gaiter must be inflated first with the patient in standing on a correctly positioned foot.
4. In the double chamber hand splint, the section covering the back of the hand must be firmly inflated first before a little air is added to the palmar section.
5. The full arm splint may be used in a therapeutic resting position for as long as one hour.
6. Splints will be removed and re-applied several times during a treatment session as the need arises to alter and adjust techniques.
7. Splints *should never be worn in direct sunlight*.
8. A cotton sleeve should be worn under the splint to protect the patient's skin against sweat rash.
9. An initial carefully positioned resting period of 20 minutes using the full arm splint should precede any exercise routine.

If the suggested programme has been followed but hand function with precision movements remains out of the patient's control it may be necessary to retrace your steps and, provided full shoulder recovery was obtained, see if full function of the elbow was really achieved. One suggestion is to return to the text given for Figure 48 and test the patient's proficiency in this exercise.

Figure 110: Rolling to propping on the affected elbow

In this figure the patient is wearing a half arm splint and sitting up forwards and sideways to rest on the ulna border of the forearm. This is a useful exercise for shoulder and elbow rehabilitation. As illustrated here the patient ought to be able to perform this exercise unaided. Lying on his back with his splinted arm placed at an angle of 45° away from his body, he lifts his head and shoulders *forwards* and sideways to rotate his upper trunk over towards the splinted arm which remains firmly on the floor. The exercise involves sitting upwards and sideways to achieve the illustrated position and lying down again *slowly*. The patient repeats the exercise for as long as his exercise tolerance allows. The *slow* movement back into the lying position is of special use in rehabilitation of the elbow. There are two necessary points to be considered:

1. The application of the half arm splint for this exercise demands that the splint is applied with the zip running down the ulna border (the inner side) of the arm, close in to the arm which becomes the weight-bearing base of the exercise. It must be positioned so as not to impede elbow bending.
2. The weight-bearing base must be correctly positioned far enough away from the patient's body to allow for a correct shoulder position when the patient moves into the propping position.

Figure 111: Elbow rehabilitation

Figure 111 shows another important elbow exercise. In the position illustrated (refer back to Fig. 14) and with the patient wearing the half arm splint, the helper is giving resistance with her right hand to the exercise he performs when he stretches his arm out straight, the upper part of his arm remaining firmly on the floor. This is the elbow movement which usually remains very weak *if it is not given special attention*. The arrow points out the direction of the movement which is suitably resisted by the helper. This must not develop into a battle of strength and the helper must let the movement happen. Her resistance will increase as the movement gets stronger. The patient's total body is positioned to ensure that overflow of muscle tone into the rest of the body will follow the weak tonal pattern.

Note that it is also important to concentrate on isolated elbow movements, e.g. with the patient seated as in Figure 81, ask him to practice *leaning firmly on the affected hand*, lean towards his affected side and bend and stretch his elbow — *pushing on the hand* to straighten the elbow. Or, as in Figure 88, leaning on the hands to straighten the elbows (but this is a less dynamic exercise). A small hand splint is often useful here.

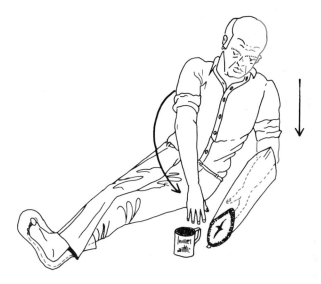

Fig. 110 Rolling to propping on the affected elbow

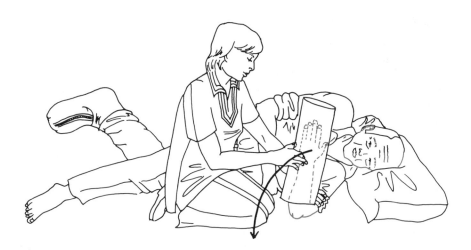

Fig. 111 Elbow rehabilitation

The small hand splint; a double chamber splint, is applied as already described with the posterior section inflated first and firmly *over the back of the hand* and then a lesser pressure applied to the anterior aspect of the hand. This is to obtain an extensor response in the fingers and this is what the whole of arm rehabilitation has been about — the need to obtain an extensor response in the fingers for final hand function. This is why it does not make sense early in the programme to test the patient's hand movement by asking him to squeeze a ball (the dominant anti-gravity flexion pattern of spasticity). Having obtained strong extension of the elbow, the patient must work to obtain the same result in the wrist and fingers.

Figure 112: Working on wrist extension

Not surprisingly, wrist extension is also a movement which frequently needs special attention. With the patient carefully positioned in the inhibiting pattern as illustrated, he practises lifting his hand backward off the table. He may use his sound hand to hold his affected forearm firmly on the table. He will almost certainly need assistance with this movement from his helper at first. The table may be turned sideways on to give a narrow surface and he may slide his arms forwards so that he leans on his forearm with his hand over the edge to give him a bigger range of movement at the wrist. He should go on practising this movement daily until he has obtained strong wrist extension.

Note that before he is able to perform this movement effectively he should be able to rotate his forearm outward so that his palm faces upward. This movement may be practised sitting at the table as illustrated with the hand splint in place. *In all of these exercises he must lean firmly on his elbow.*

Figure 113: Working on finger extension

The hand splint may be positioned as illustrated in Figure 113. Then, as illustrated in Figure 112 but with the cantilever table turned side on, the patient leans on his forearms with his fingers extended over the edge of the table. He may hold his affected thumb in position with his sound hand while he practises bending and stretching his proximal knuckle joints moving straight fingers downwards and upwards. The upward movement of the fingers — or full extension of the fingers — *must be re-educated.* At the end of this exercise he should stand up with the splint removed and practise leaning on the table on his finger-tips taking his weight through straight fingers.

Figures 110–113 give helpful suggestions towards obtaining a working, functional hand with precision movements.

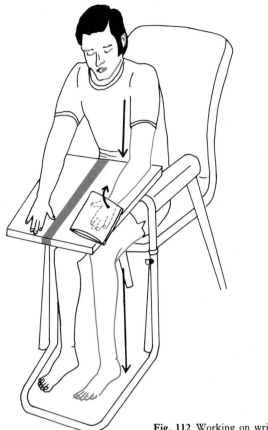

Fig. 112 Working on wrist extension

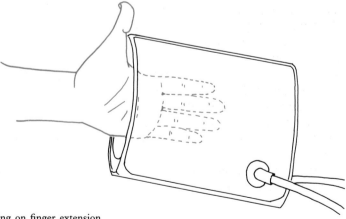

Fig. 113 Working on finger extension

Summing up

Successful rehabilitation as presented here depends on the physiotherapist and her ability to understand the basic problems that face the stroke patient. She must be able to assess the patient's needs, she must be ready to interpret sound principles of treatment into a sound and realistic physical programme which will lead towards controlled movement and recovery — the optimum recovery for the individual patient. Particularly where full recovery is not possible, a fair chance of reasonable recovery of function ought to be offered. As presented here, this chance will be given. The physiotherapist *must make a cheerful and hopeful approach*, assess each patient individually and find ways and means of getting round any other difficulties that may be present, especially in the elderly patient. Above all, she must be ready to assess the patient's family and, wherever possible, to teach and to hand over care to the family who may continue to be guided by her skill. This skill must include the necessary knowledge to make sound decisions which must also include withdrawal of her support at the right time, leaving her patient in the semi-skilled home care which she has first established. Above all, the physiotherapist must have the backing of the patient's doctor and the support of any other social services that may be required.

This book has been written to bring understanding to all who undertake the home care of a stroke patient. Consequently it is written in lay language which should be readily understood by all. Because it is intended as a guide to physical handling, and not as a complete treatment manual, there are many stroke problems that are not mentioned. There is no place for them here. Other problems must be the business of the expert and the expert must be asked for advice. But many of *these problems are caused, or built-up, by bad handling* which leads to the patient's failure to *live in the pattern of recovery*. Thus it will be understood how great is the need to shed the light of understanding on the day to day handling of the stroke patient. The urgent need to start correct positioning from day one after onset of the stroke must mean there is an urgent need to educate the families involved. It is hoped the expert will assess the family and, where possible, introduce the suitable caring member to this book. The expert and the family member will then quickly reach a common understanding and the expert will withdraw while the home team takes over. The withdrawal will take place as quickly — or as slowly — as circumstances dictate but, wherever possible, it is essential to give the home team some support, be it only by telephone. Any further difficulties that may arise which lead to further questions must be turned over to the expert. Finally, there is one question which sometimes arises and which ought not to arise if the home helper has fully understood what it means for her patient to *live in the pattern of recovery*. The question is:

Why not give the patient a calliper to support the weak leg?

If you, the reader, ask this question now, having decided you understand all that is written in these pages, the book has failed sadly in the object it set out to achieve.

So, why not give him a calliper? Would he not learn to stand and walk much more quickly if he stood with a calliper firmly supporting his weak knee? Yes, he would stand more quickly, and he would walk more quickly — after a fashion! He would stand, but he would stand on the front part of his foot — a wrongly positioned base. This pressure through the front part of his foot, instead of inhibiting the unwanted reflexes, would at once lead to a build-up of these unwanted reflexes and the patient would begin propping on a leg held stiffly in extension — the complete pattern of spasticity (Fig. 7) — and the first aim of all treatment is to prevent spasticity. This would in turn lead to walking in the pattern of spasticity; the hip would turn outwards, it would be drawn backwards and it would quickly stiffen up in this position. Inevitably the patient would use his leg as a prop and move if forwards by swinging his foot in an awkward arc; he would never again weight-bear over a correctly positioned foot, and he would continue to build-up leg spasticity which would put an end to any hope of ever regaining a properly functioning leg.

Try this for yourself. Try standing with both your knees fully braced back. Maintain this position with one leg while you take a step forward with the other. What happens? As you transfer your weight forward the supporting leg takes all the weight and, if you continue to keep the knee quite straight, all your weight goes through the front part of the supporting foot. This is exactly what happens when a knee is tightly supported in the straight position by a calliper. In normal walking the support knee is always slightly bent — much time is spent in teaching the stroke patient to weight-bear over a semi-bent knee as has been shown (e.g. Figs 88, 89 and 107.).

If you are tempted to ask the question — why not a calliper? — turn back to the notes given for Figure 21 and see if this was properly understood. Then, if you still believe you are able to help the stroke patient who is to be cared for at home, it would be wise to go right back to the beginning of the book and study it all over again. After that you may find it becomes a helpful and reliable guide.

Successful home rehabilitation for the stroke patient has become an urgent necessity. More and more stroke patients are being cared for at home and hospital facilities are not increasing. Beside this, the home background, with its familiar surroundings and known and loved faces, is considered in many cases to be the best place for the patient to recover and to rehabilitate successfully. We must spread our knowledge and, wherever possible, the lay person must become involved. 'Wisdom is the principal thing; therefore get wisdom; and with all thy getting get understanding.'

By the very nature of the undertaking, *stroke rehabilitation is not a subject to be left solely to the expert*; it must be understood and undertaken by all those who come into daily contact with the patient so that they make it possible for him to *live in a pattern*. It is this simple pattern for living which is at the heart of all true stroke rehabilitation and which leads to the optimum recovery for each individual patient.

In this book it has been shown that this pattern for daily living is built round positioning, and positioning has been described in detail. It has been shown to include all attitudes in lying, sitting, or standing and all advancing progressions from one to the next. It has also been shown that this vital need for positioning must include any part of the body which is used to bear weight because the position of this weight-bearing base directly affects the position of the limb or body above it. It has also been shown that weight-bearing plays a most important part in recovery and is, therefore, an essential part of rehabilitation.

The reasoning behind:

1. Positioning
2. The need to weight- bear
3. The need to increase sensory stimulation by touch (including deep pressure), use of the eyes (including the use of a mirror) and use of hearing (including firm, simple commands)

has been clearly stated.

If any part of the book gives the reader difficulty because of failure to understand it, it has been suggested that the expert in stroke rehabilitation should be consulted. Only with understanding will correct methods be used. It has also been urgently suggested that, wherever possible, the patient himself should be taught the reasoning behind positioning so that the care of his own limbs may be handed over to him, even if he needs constant reminders to stay within the pattern until it becomes an accustomed, and therefore almost an automatic, way of life.

What supporting services are available?

These may be grouped under three headings:

1. *Health Services may provide:*

Home nursing
Health visiting
Special nursing equipment, e.g. incontinance pads

2. *Social Services may provide:*

Adaptations to the home
Home helps
Aids to daily living, e.g. Rollator walking aid

3. *Department of Health and Social Security may provide*:

Financial help

4. *Chest, Heart and Stroke Association*

Provides back-up support and offers two very useful booklets which may help to answer any other questions:

Stroke, a handbook for the patient's family by Graham Mulley MB, ChB, MRCP

Stroke illness, twenty questions and the answers.

Both are available from the above association at Tavistock House North, Tavistock Square, London WC1H 9JE.

7

Case histories

Three brief case histories of progress made after the onset of severe disability caused by stroke will now be given. They are illustrated by a series of photographs showing *some* of the key positions and the advancing stages of returning function. It must be stressed that it has not been possible to include all the stages of rehabilitation; this would involve many more pictures which could run into a volume on their own. It was decided, when considering the use of a series of photographs to illustrate this book, that the progress made by a male patient should be covered as the text refers to the patient as 'he'. However, even this one patient could have had many more pictures to illustrate his progress if every stage of his rehabilitation were to be shown. In other words, by all means use the photographs as a guide *but* do not forget to follow the stage by stage diagrams which accompany the text of the book. Note, also, that the male patient in the photographs, Mr G., had right- sided disability, as did Mrs R., while Miss A. was left- sided.

It should also be emphasised that these three patients were not handpicked because they were expected to do well — far from it. Miss A.'s outlook at the beginning of rehabilitation was very poor and she far surpassed even my best hopes for her. Viewed in retrospect, I feel it would be fair to say that these three patients are fairly typical of many others that have passed through my hands and have been treated along the lines suggested in this book.

Mr G.

Mr G., not yet a senior citizen, was admitted to the hospital rehabilitation unit where I worked in February 1977. He had suffered a fairly severe stroke early in the previous month and had been admitted to a general hospital. On admission to our unit as an in-patient we found he had *right-sided paralysis* and slurring of his speech. We decided to take a series of photographs of his rehabilitation. It was thought that his progress might be used to demonstrate to other stroke victims the pattern his rehabilitation followed. Prior to his stroke his left hand had been dominant.

If all the stages of rehabilitation were shown, the photographs involved would need a book to themselves, so it was decided to include a few of the

180

key positions as a guide to the course his treatment followed. Suffice it to say that his rehabilitation exactly followed the lines suggested in this book. But, it should be noted that he had *right-sided* disability, not left-sided as in the diagrams illustrating the text of the book.

On admission he was very carefully assessed both medically and physically and it was decided that his exercise tolerance *at that time* was not good. Nevertheless, it was decided to push on with a full rehabilitation programme but to give him frequent resting periods during treatment sessions and these were given with meticulous positioning in lying. Tests also showed that he had loss of body image. This means that he was not properly relating his affected limbs to the rest of his body. Pressure techiques were used to assist recovery of lost body image and also because there was already strong evidence of the onset of spasticity.

He progressed as we hoped, and, after four weeks, his wife readily agreed to become involved in his treatment. She came dressed in slacks two afternoons a week to join him in exercise sessions on the floor mat. She was carefully instructed in the techniques we use.

By the beginning of May, approximately three months after admission to our rehabilitation unit, he had returned home where his wife helped him to continue with careful positioning and the advancing exercise routines as set out in this book. A relative brought him to us by car once a week to continue exercise routines under our supervision. His wife also continued to attend to him, and to be completely involved in the recovery programme. His speech difficulty resolved fairly quickly. The photographs show the physical progress he made.

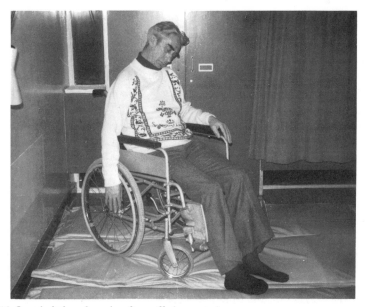

Fig. 114 On admission, 3 weeks after suffering a stroke.

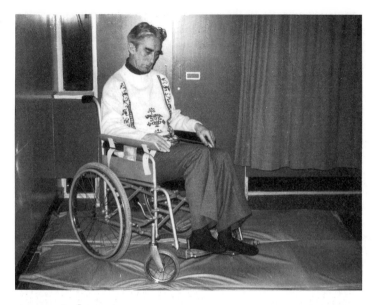

Fig. 115 Meticulous positioning was started at once as was training in sitting balance. Note the gutter arm rest.

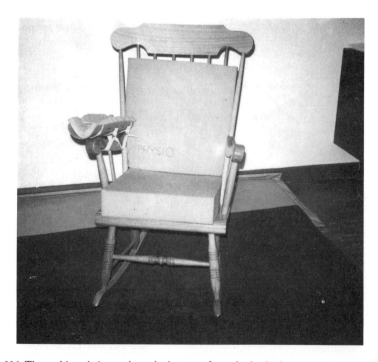

Fig. 116 The rocking chair was brought into use from the beginning.

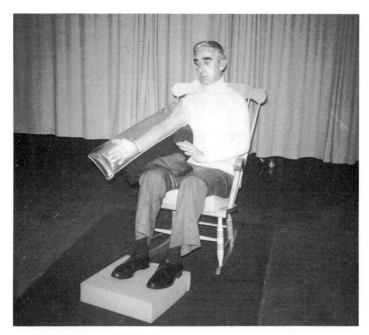

Fig. 117 Using the rocking chair and a pressure splint to position his affected arm and help to make him aware of it.

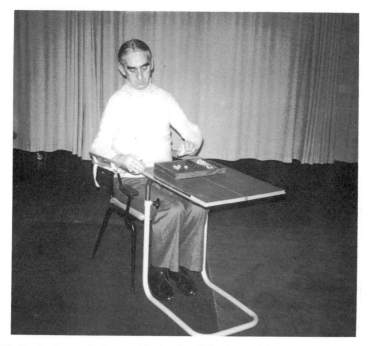

Fig. 118 Continuing meticulous positioning for all daytime activity — living in the pattern.

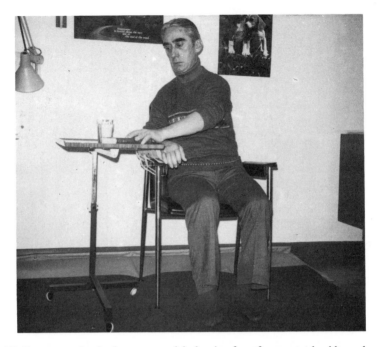

Fig. 119 Forearm resting in the gutter, weight-bearing from forearm to shoulder as he turns to reach for a glass of water.

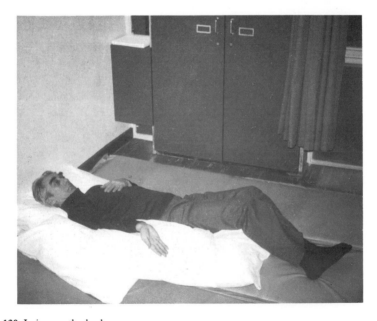

Fig. 120 Lying on the back.

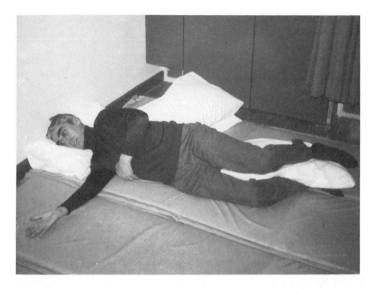

Fig. 121 Lying on the affected side.

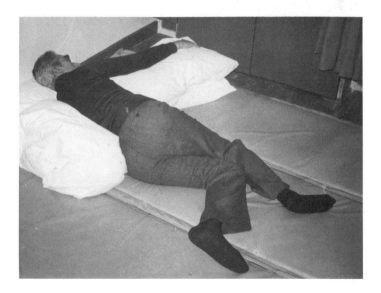

Fig. 122 Lying on the sound side.

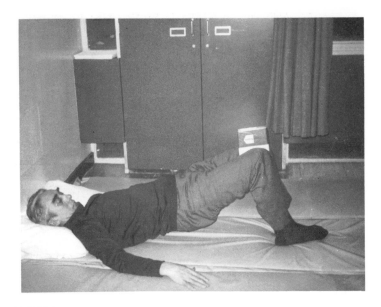

Fig. 123 Bridging.

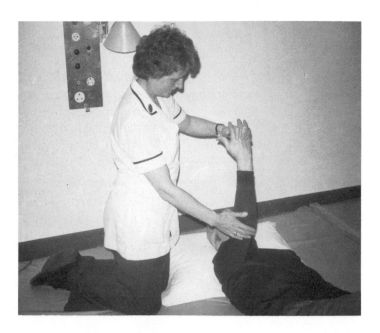

Fig. 124 Arm raising with external rotation.

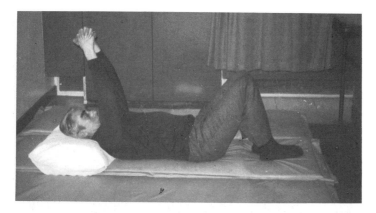

Fig. 125 Arm raising — self-care.

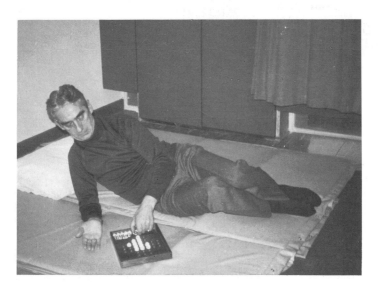

Fig. 126 Rolling to elbow propping.

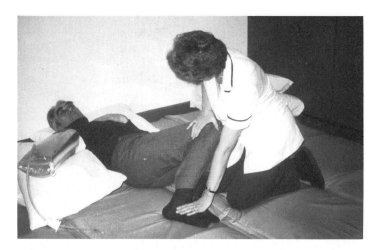

Fig. 127 Arm positioned in splint, hip rolling.

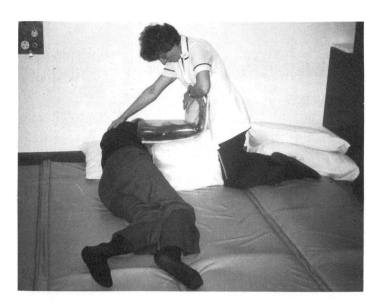

Fig. 128 Weight-bearing from hand to shoulder, using pressure splint support.

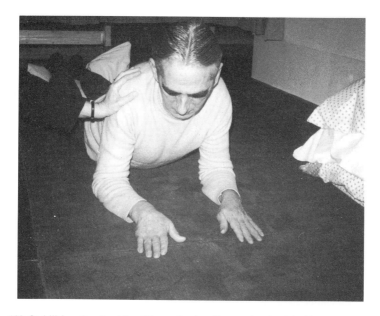

Fig. 129 Stabilising the shoulder. The patient's wife now involved in his treatment.

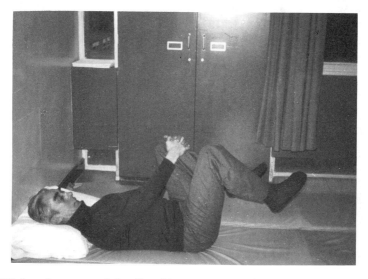

Fig. 130 Learning to control the affected leg.

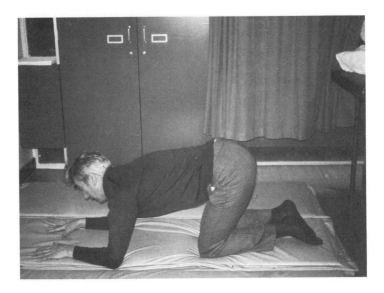

Fig. 131 Crawling position with forearm propping.

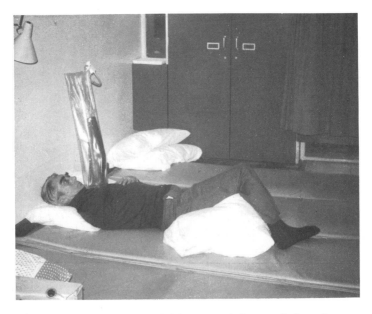

Fig. 132 After much hard work, he holds his arm steady in space (splint on).

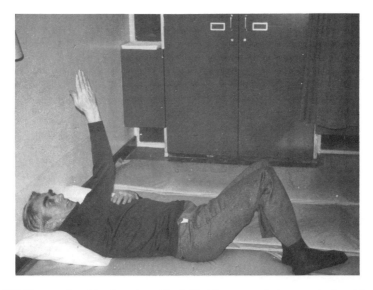

Fig. 133 More weeks of hard work and he holds his arm steady in space (splint off).

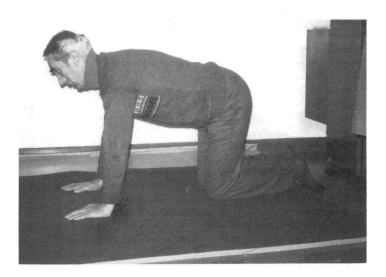

Fig. 134 Full crawling position is finally established with elbow stability.

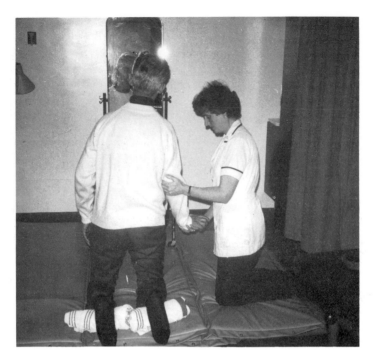

Fig. 135 Learning to balance, or stabilise, in stand kneeling with help of mirror. Supported on his affected side and transferring his weight over his affected hip.

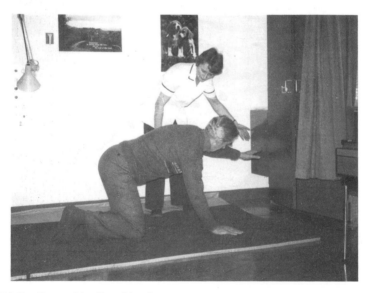

Fig. 136 Standing on his affected hand.

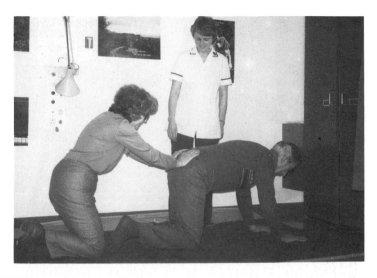

Fig. 137 His wife takes part: 'Don't let me push you'. Pressure must be gentle, built up slowly, and must be withdrawn slowly.

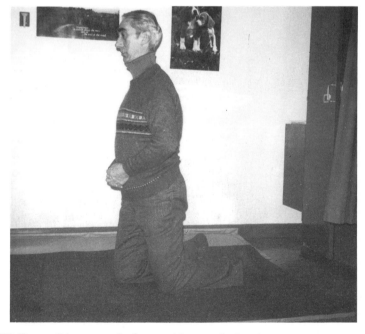

Fig. 138 Knee walking across the floor straight towards the mirror.

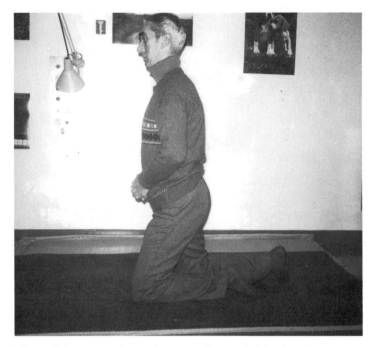

Fig. 139 Controlled posture as he continues to walk towards his mirror image.

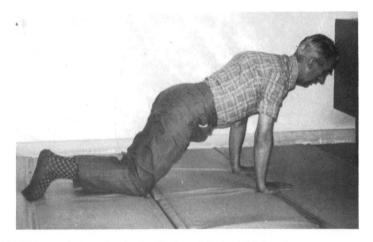

Fig. 140 This was the exercise that he felt 'gave him back his hand'.

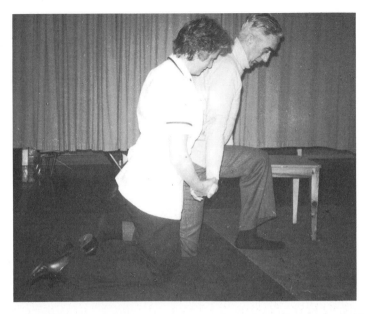

Fig. 141 Getting up from the floor. Sound hand on the stool, standing on the sound foot.

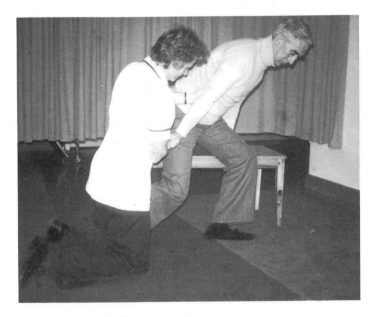

Fig. 142 Getting up from the floor — second stage.

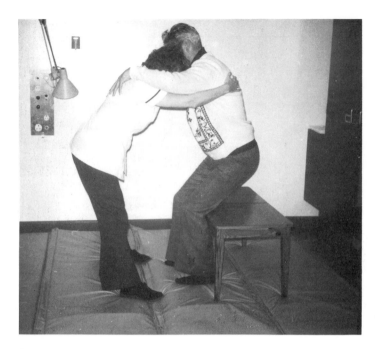

Fig. 143 Learning to stand up from sitting.

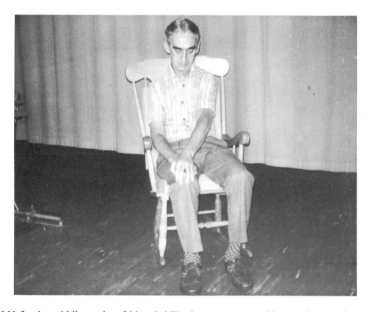

Fig. 144 In the middle weeks of his rehabilitation programme this was the exercise he found most useful for his leg — using the rocking chair with extra pressure from the knee to heel.

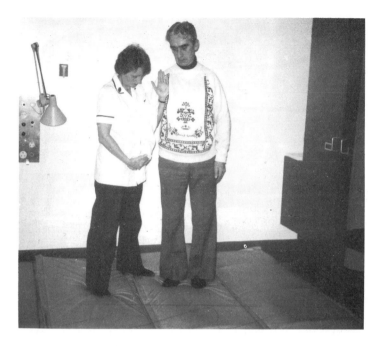

Fig. 145 Learning to stabilise in standing and to transfer weight over the affected leg.

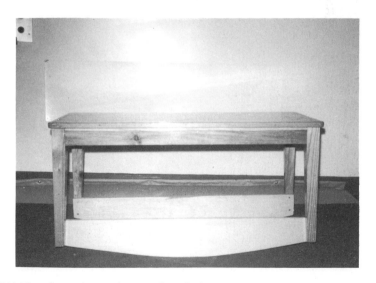

Fig. 146 Next the stool on rockers was brought into use.

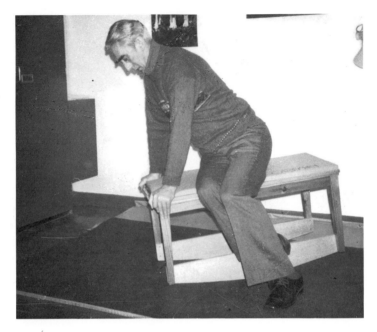

Fig. 147 Rocking to 'stand' on the affected hand.

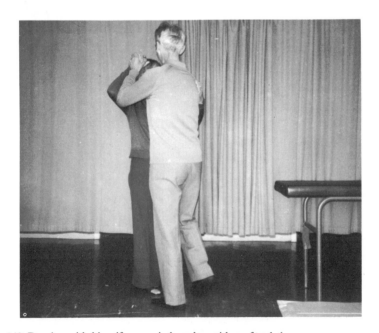

Fig. 148 Dancing with his wife — a circle waltz, with perfect balance.

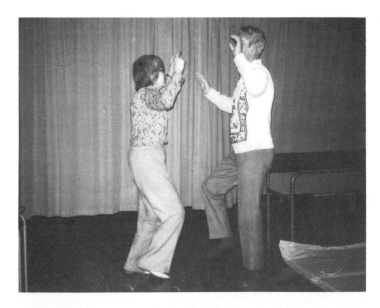

Fig. 149 More ambitious — dancing a Highland Fling.

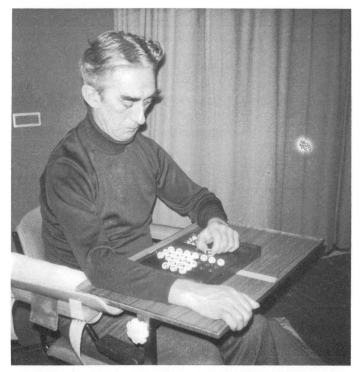

Fig. 150 In the final stages of rehabilitation he could use either hand for small precision movements but he still automatically positioned his affected arm when he used his sound hand.

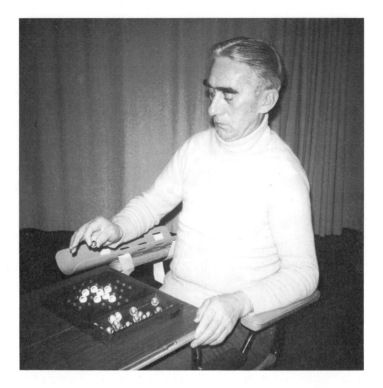

Fig. 151 Affected hand now fully rehabilitated and used for precision movement.

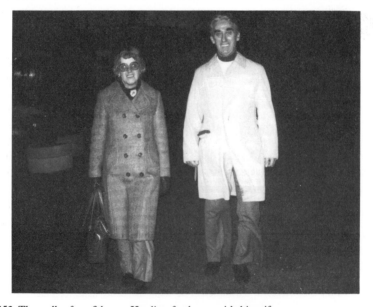

Fig. 152 The walk of confidence. Heading for home with his wife.

Miss A.

Miss A. is a delightful lady approaching her 80th birthday. She came into my care in our rehabilitation unit at the end of June 1977. She had spent two months in another hospital and was sent to us with a written request which read: 'If you achieve any improvement here, please let us know how you did it.' She was in a bad way because she had very severe sensory loss. She appeared to neglect her left side totally and to have no idea where her affected limbs were. Indeed, she did not seem aware that her left limbs were completely paralysed. As we expected, tests showed that she was quite unaware of the left side of her body. With our worst fears confirmed, we did not expect her to make much progress in rehabilitation because of her extreme degree of sensory loss. She had no sitting balance and was quite incapable of standing unless she was held upright by two people.

We set out to give intensive treatment. This included all the techniques set out in this book and we also added a lengthy daily session of intermittent pressure to the affected limbs. This is done by using a special mechanical pump and special splints to give fluctuating deep pressure and must be done by the expert. It stimulates the sensory nerves and would not be given where spasticity — or too much muscle tone — is a problem. Intensive treatment for Miss A. also included frequent resting periods between exercises with careful positioning, the use of sustained pressure splints with exercises as described in this book, and stage by stage establishment of stability in the key positions of rolling to *propping* to *kneeling* to *crawling* to *standing*. All the techniques suggested in this book were used, and used in the correct sequence of motor development patterns. We knew that motor development and sensory development must go forward together if Miss A. was to have any hope of recovery. We knew we had time to give the required treatment because it was expected that she would not rehabilitate sufficiently to go home and she could expect to face long term care in an institution. There are long waiting lists for such places and so time was on our side.

Meanwhile, Miss A. showed a cheerful disposition, a dogged determination to get better and go home. Nothing could deflect her from this fixed purpose. She frequently insisted that she intended to go home to her own flat. She lives alone in a tenement building at the top of a spiral staircase. The banister is on the narrow side of the stairs, right hand side going up. She made the following progress:

After 4 months: she was still neglecting the left arm but had achieved good stability in sitting. She had learnt to roll, to roll over to prop on her forearms and was well stabilised in this position.

After 5 months: she had established balance in the crawling position provided the physiotherapist gave support to her affected elbow.

After 7 months: she had established balance in stand kneeling with her hands clasped at her front. Her knee control was still poor and she still needed constant reminders to *watch* her limbs, to *move slowly* and to *concencrate*.

After 8 months: she had established balanced walking in stand kneeling and was having daily training sessions in stabilising in standing. Standing balance was proving difficult to achieve. The occupational therapist began intensive work, paying particular attention to her neglect of her left arm.

After 10 months: she no longer neglected the left arm and had begun to walk independently on the Rollator Aid. It began to look as if she might go home. She was taken by the physio and occupational therapists to visit her home. An alarming staircase! But once she got up into her flat she was very happy and very much 'at home' in her own surroundings. Her flat seemed very much in need of electrical rewiring and an electrician later confirmed this. It was decided she would continue her rehabilitation programme in hospital, now with the definite hope that she might soon go home.

During the 11th month: she began practising stair climbing crabwise in the way she would have to do it to negotiate the narrow side of a spiral. She was still neglecting her left foot. It was now 11 months since the onset of her stroke and she had spent 8 months in our care. The rewiring of her flat was undertaken at her own expense and took 3 months to complete. Approximately a year after her admission to our unit she was discharged home to live quite safely alone with the support of a daily home help, plus some very good long-standing friends, and she was content. She had back-up services *but* she was successfully living alone. Very soon she tackled the spiral staircase and went out shopping! The following Christmas she flew to Holland to visit her nearest relations. She sent us this message written by herself on a post card:

> 'Here I am enjoying my holiday with relatives. Christmas here very different from Scotland. Weather seasonable, canals frozen and almost everybody on skates (except me). Thank you very much for making this holiday come true for me. Hope you have a good Xmas and I wish you a very happy New Year.'

I must add, *we* did not make the holiday she dreamed of come true. We could have done nothing without her cheerful spirit and her determination to get back to normal living.

I regret that I did not take photographs to cover her months of rehabilitation and demonstrate her progress. I took four pictures to show the end result of her treatment and two to show the simple fitments that were all that was needed to make independent living in her own home a relatively simple matter.

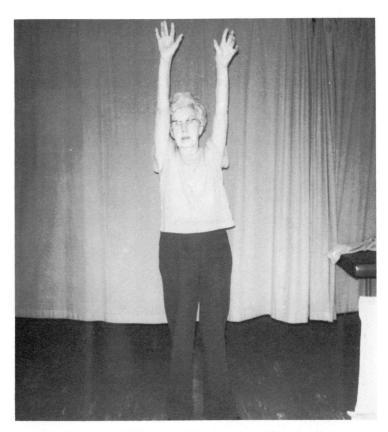

Fig. 153 'Look what I can do!' The successful end to a year of hard work.

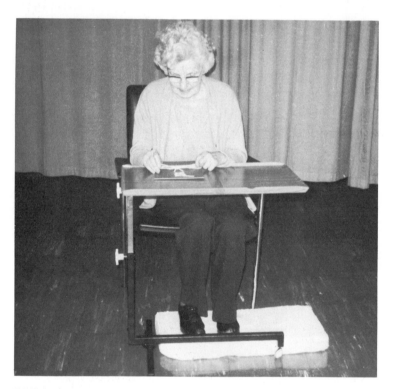

Fig. 154 Tying a bow.

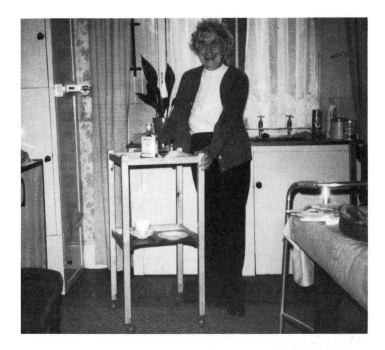

Fig. 155 Home at last! Cheerful hospitality offered to a visitor. The trolley is a very useful rehabilitation aid.

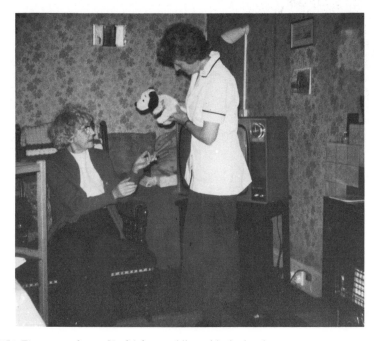

Fig. 156 The very soft toy. Useful for moulding with the hands.

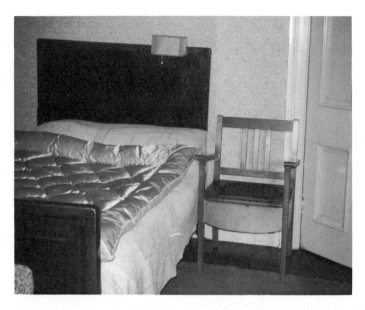

Fig. 157 The bedside commode suitably placed in position for the left-sided stroke. For the right-sided stroke it would be placed on the other side of the bed.

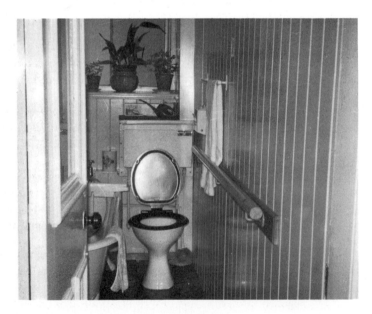

Fig. 158 A hand-rail was added to the bathroom wall.

Mrs R.

Mrs R., a charming senior citizen, came into my care at the end of April 1978. The date of onset of her stroke was seven weeks earlier and she was admitted for the care of our rehabilitation team from another hospital. On admission she was found to have a rigid right leg thrust out in full extensor spasticity, severe flexion spasm in the right arm with the shoulder fixed in internal rotation and she had no stability in standing. After careful assessment the following note was entered on her physiotherapy treatment card: 'Problem — severe spasticity developing fast after recent onset of stroke but sensory loss does not appear to be present. Exercise tolerance: treat with care.'

Ten days later it was noted that:

> 'She is responding well to long periods in the rocking chair with careful positioning. Her leg is much less rigid. Her arm is also improving, responding well to careful positioning and pressure techniques with the sustained pressure splint. She is now standing and stabilising well with the help of the Zimmer Aid. Outlook for early discharge home is good. Her husband has been asked to join in the treatment sessions. Has now begun (and is working with) rolling and propping routines on the floor interspaced with frequent rest periods with careful positioning.'

Within 2 weeks the necessary members of the rehabilitation team took her to visit her home. Again all went well and it was thought that the back entrance to the house was the one she should use, in spite of a very deep step at the back door. The front approach had a very narrow path and very awkward steps. The house itself appeared to need minimal adaptations apart from adding toilet rails and a bath seat. She was sent home to continue rehabilitation there exactly five weeks after her admission to our care and I followed up with minimal home supervison for another month — approximately one visit a week.

Her family took care of everything. As well as becoming head cook and bottle washer, her husband helped her to continue with careful positioning and home exercises.

When asked at the end of rehabilitation which exercise she felt had been of most help she did not hesitate with her answer. 'Undoubtedly the rocking chair.' She had been taught to use it when she first came to us with her affected arm carefully positioned in a pressure splint and her feet placed on non- slip foam rubber cushioning so that she rocked by **pushing on her heels**. Later she used it as illustrated in the photographs. The photographs show continuing care at home and are presented here to underline the part that can be played in rehabilitation by the caring family member.

It is important to remember that, *without meticulous positioning and correct retraining of controlled movement*, the severe spasticity this patient already showed when she came into our care would have taken her over. She would have remained a helpless cripple for the rest of her life and she would not have gone home because it would have been beyond her husband's strength to lift her about. It is also important to remember that her rehabilitation was not slowed down by the extra disability of sensory loss. Had it been, her time spent in hospital would have been considerably longer. Towards the end of the year she ventured out to a dinner dance with her husband.

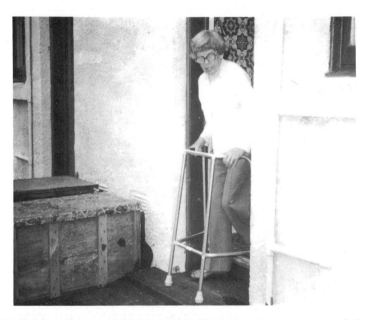

Fig. 159 Zimmer Aid to go out into the garden. The two wooden steps were made by the family, wide enough to accommodate the Zimmer.

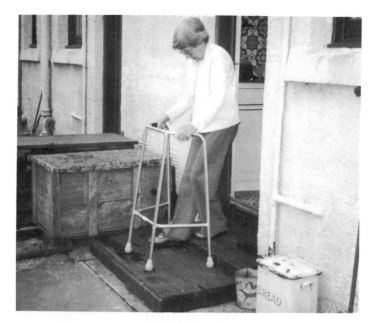

Fig. 160 Deep step successfully negotiated. A hand-rail was installed 3 weeks later and the Zimmer discarded.

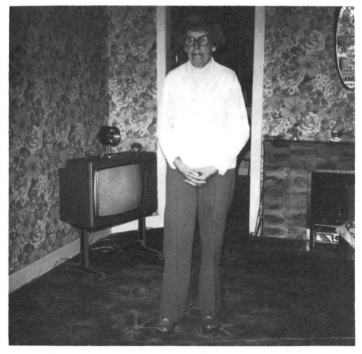

Fig. 161 Beginning to walk alone.

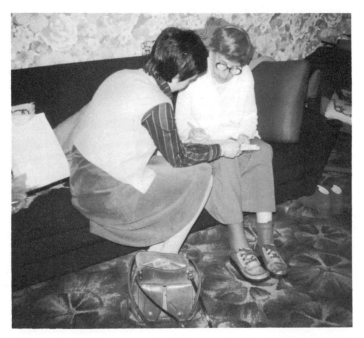

Fig. 162 The speech therapist uncovered a hidden speech difficulty which was causing some distress.

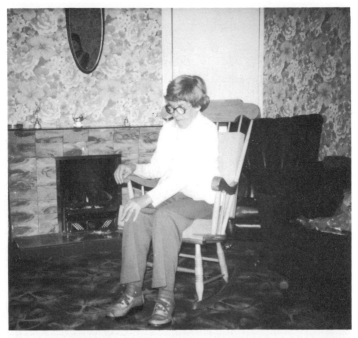

Fig. 163 Using the rocking-chair to assist arm and leg recovery. Weight-bearing from elbow to shoulder and heel to knee.

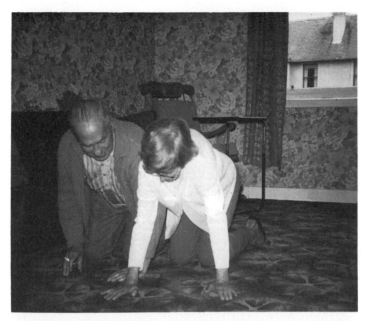

Fig. 164 Crawling. Family involvement as the patient is encouraged to lean towards her husband who crawls on her affected side.

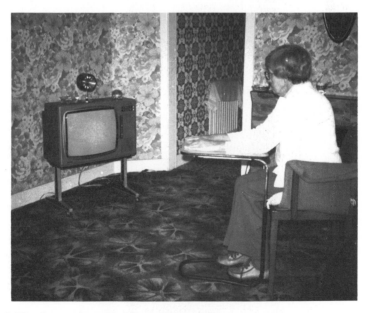

Fig. 165 The therapeutic position for watching television.

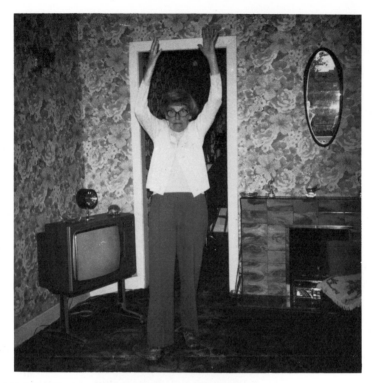

Fig. 166 Rehabilitation continues to move in the right direction.

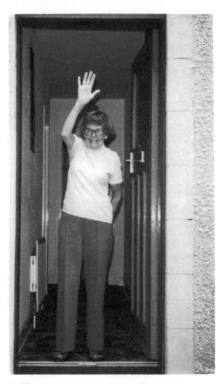

Fig. 167 A final farewell. Waving good-bye with the 'stroke' hand, and with the satisfied smile of successful rehabilitation.

Glossary

Some words which may be used about the patient:

Agnosia	A perceptual disturbance giving difficulty in recognition. Failure to recognise.
Associated reactions	These occur with all attempted movements and are released postural reactions deprived of voluntary control because of brain damage. They give a widespread increase of spasticity if the limbs are not inhibited.
Body image	The image in an individual's mind of his own body.
Cognition	Knowing, or awareness, in the widest sense, including sensation, perception etc.
Dysarthria	A disorder of speech which includes difficulty in articulation due to motor defect in the muscles of lips, tongue, palate, throat.
Dysphasia	A disorder of language which may, or may not, include difficulty in comprehension. More usually, comprehension remains intact.
Hemianopia	Blindness in one half of the visual field of one or both eyes. (A defect which usually clears up fairly quickly.)
Muscle tone	A state of slight tension of muscle fibres when not in use which enables them to respond more swiftly to a stimulus.
Positioning	Placing in the optimum position to allow for, and promote, recovery.
Primitive movement	Movement which is entirely reflex in character, fundamental, belonging to the beginning.
Prognosis	Forecasting, or forecast, especially of the course of a disease.
Recovery pattern	The position, or the pattern of movement, which inhibits spasticity to allow for, and promote, recovery.
Rehabilitation	Obtaining the maximum degree of physical and psychological independence after disability by means

of a careful planned physical programme which must be presented to the patient with cheerful optimism, an optimistic approach being a necessary part of successful rehabilitation.

Spatial orientation   Awareness of body position in relation to space.

Ulna   The inner and larger of the two bones of the forearm. Ulna border, the inner border.

Visual agnosia   Failure to interpret what is seen. This type of 'blindness' usually clears up more slowly than hemianopia.

Appendix

SOME USEFUL ADDRESSES

Pressure splints

Urias: Orally Inflatable Air Splints (for sustained pressure) Made in Denmark by Svend Andersen Plastic Industri A/S, DK4652 Haarlev, Denmark.
Apply to the Danish address for the address of your local distributor.
Distributor for Scotland: Whitefield (Medical) Ltd 10 Ardmillan Place, Edinburgh EH11 2JR U.K.

Therapeutic putty (for final stage of hand rehabilitation)

Carter's Therapeutic Putty supplied by Carter's, Alfred Street, Westbury, Wilts., U.K.

The suggested rocking chair

A do-it-yourself kit from any branch of Timberland, U.K.

A new arm support

The Steed cushion — positions and supports the affected arm with the patient in sitting in the early days.
Particulars from:
Nottingham Rehab., 17 Ludlow Hill Road, Melton Road, West Bridgford, Nottingham NG2 6HD.

Suggested further reading

The Stroke Patient: A team approach, 3rd edn by Margaret Johnstone. Churchill Livingstone, Edinburgh

The Chest, Heart and Stroke Association offers two very useful booklets which may help to answer any other questions:

1. *Stroke*, a handbook for the patient's family by Graham Mulley
2. *Stroke illness*, twenty questions and the answers.

Both are available from the Association at Tavistock House North, Tavistock Square, London WC1H 9JE.

Index

Anti-gravity muscles, 20, 40
Anti-spasticity pattern, 20–22

Ball, misuse of, 118
Body alignment, 46

Calliper, 80, 176–177
Cerebral haemorrhage, 2
Cerebral thrombosis, 2
Cognition, 6
Communication, 65–78
  charts, 77
Conscious recognition, 5
Constipation, 7
Controlled movement, 9

Dehydration, 3, 38
Dentures, 76
Depression, 1, 6–7
Developing spasticity 16–17
Dysarthria, 6, 66, 75
Dysphasia, 6, 66
Dyspraxia, 66, 73

Emotion, 6
Expressive dysphasia, 71

Footboard, 35, 38
Footstool, 60, 61
Furniture positioning, 23–24

Getting out of bed, 42–49
Gutter arm-rest, 52–53

Haemorrhage, cerebral, 2
Hand clasp, 34, 92, 94
Hearing aids, 76
Heel, of foot, 61–62
  of hand, 61–62
Hemiparesis, 5
Hemiplegia, 5
Hypertension, 2

Incontinence, 7

Knee control, 136, 142, 162
Kneeling in crawling, 106
  in stand kneeling, 106

Living in pattern, 61–62, 79–82

Mirror, use of, 46, 51
Motor development, 10
Movement, controlled, 10
  primitive, 10–15

Normal development 10

Optimism, 42

Pain, shoulder, 32, 45, 82
Positioning, furniture, 23–24
  patient, 23–64
  weight-bearing, 61–62
Pressure splint, arm, 147–155
Primitive reflex movement, 9, 10, 13, 15

Receptive dysphasia, 67
Recovery pattern, 20–22, 79–82
Reflex movement, 10–15
Rehabilitation, 1, 9, 79

Self-care, 1, 19, 34, 124–125
Sensory loss, 13, 16, 41, 201
Sex life, 6
Shoulder care, 32–34, 150
  pain, 32, 45, 88
  pain prevention, 88, 100, 104
  positioning, 20–22
Smoking, 2
Spasticity, 16–22
  prevention, 20, 147, 170
Speech therapy, 65–77
Stabilising, 84, 122
  in crawling, 106, 158
  in elbow propping, 86, 88

Stabilising, (cont'd)
  in side-lying, 84
  in sitting, 48, 122
  in stand kneeling, 106
  in standing, 140
Stroke, what is?, 1
  cause, 2, 3
Supporting services, 178–179

Thrombosis, cerebral, 2
Training sitting balance, 48–49,
  122

Walking aids, 138
Weight-bearing base, 60–63
Word-finding difficulty, 71

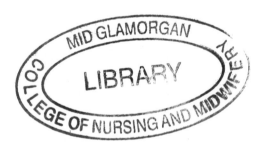